homeopathy

the practical guide
for the 21st century

Beth MacEoin

homeopathy

the practical guide for the 21st century

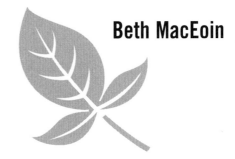

Beth MacEoin

Kyle Cathie Limited

Senior Editor **Caroline Taggart**
Editor **Vicki Murrell**
Design **Mark Latter, Pink Stripe Design**
Proofreader **Elaine Koster**
Indexer **Alex Corrin**
Production **Sha Huxtable and Alice Holloway**

First published in Great Britain in 2006 by Kyle Cathie Limited
122 Arlington Road, London NW1 7HP
general.enquiries@kyle-cathie.com
www.kylecathie.com

ISBN 1 85626 609 5
ISBN (13-digit) 1 85626 609 3

10 9 8 7 6 5 4 3 2 1

Printed and Bound in Singapore by Tien-Wah Press

Disclaimer

**The contents of this book are for information only and are intended to assist readers in identifying
symptoms and conditions they may be experiencing. The book is not intended to be a substitute for taking
proper medical advice and should not be relied upon in this way. Always consult a qualified doctor or health
practitioner. The author and publisher cannot accept responsibility for illness arising out of the failure to
seek medical advice from a doctor.**

contents

foreword

Homeopathy is one of the most flexible, user-friendly and effective forms of complementary medicine available to us and yet many people feel unsure about how to use it successfully at home. In every high street pharmacy there are shelves and shelves of homeopathic medicines on prominent display along with a host of other tantilising complementary products and yet, while they may look intriguing as they sit there in their high-tech, one-click-dispenser containers (all very twenty-first century), what on earth are we actually expected to do with them?

If this sounds familiar, then this book has been written especially with you in mind as my aim throughout has been to pack into this single, easy-to-use volume all the essential information you need in order to use homeopathy confidently and effectively at home, both for yourself and for your family.

I can't emphasise enough how practical this guide has been designed to be. If you have a health problem, you need to be able to treat it with the minimum of fuss, hitting on the homeopathic solution as quickly and accurately as possible. This book will not expect or encourage you to work like a homeopathic practitioner in embryo, nor will it give endless detail about the historical development of homeopathy as a medical science. Instead it will give you everything you need to know about safe, first-aid, acute prescribing at home.

Once you know how to take down a patient's symptom picture it will be a trouble-free task to identify the correct homeopathic solution as all you have to do is glance at the quick-reference tables given for each condition so that you can assess which remedy fits your particular situation most closely. And with each case there are clear guidelines so you will be able to recognise immediately if a situation has passed outside the remit of home prescribing and needs emergency help or conventional medical advice.

Homeopathy can also be very effectively supported by many kinds of complementary treatment, such as essential oils, herbal medicines and good nutrition. This book therefore places homeopathic self-prescribing within a working context, showing how it relates to other forms of treatment, as well as conventional medicine, and how it can be used to deal with a whole host of common family traumas in the most comprehensive, gentle way that works with the body rather than against it.

homeopathy in a nutshell

This chapter cuts through the mystique of homeopathic theory by concentrating on the absolute essentials you need to know in order to be able to use this book effectively.

what is homeopathy?

Homeopathy is a gentle, holistic system of medicine that uses highly dilute substances to stimulate the body's potential for self-healing. Whereas conventional medicines work by suppressing symptoms, homeopathic medicines are selected to work with them in order to let the body free itself of illness. The idea behind this is simple but very effective: a substance that causes a particular illness or symptoms in a healthy person will modify or cure the same illness or symptom in a sick one. Medicines are therefore selected on the basis of their similarity to the patient's symptoms in line with the fundamental homeopathic principle of 'like cures like'.

Homeopathy was developed by a German doctor called Samuel Hahnemann approximately two hundred years ago. Trained as a conventional doctor, Hahnemann became horrified by the side-effects of orthodox drugs and procedures that he witnessed in the patients he was trying to help. In an effort to restore his patients to good health with the minimum risk of distress through toxic side-effects, Hahnemann started to research the healing powers of natural remedies, systematically testing individual substances on his own healthy constitution and that of his family and friends in order to record their exact and specific effect. In this way he collated a detailed 'symptom picture' for each remedy and published his findings between 1811 and 1821 in the six volumes of his *Materia Medica Pura*.

With all this research, Hahnemann developed his homeopathic practice on the principle that if he correctly matched a symptom picture to its compatible remedy then the patient would be swiftly restored to health. However, on many an occasion, the patient's symptoms actually got worse before they got better and so Hahnemann began to dilute the remedy in order to temper its aggravating effect on the body.

Although the extremely dilute nature of homeopathic medicine leads to some scepticism about how these remedies can possibly work, tentative steps have been made towards an explanation. One approach involves the 'memory of water' theory, which suggests that the water solution acts as a sort of polymer or liquid crystal and holds the imprint or memory of the original starting material. When a sufficient match exists between the main symptoms of a patient and the key features of the administered homeopathic remedy, it kick-starts the body's self-healing mechanism so that the symptoms are resolved by the body's own defences.

Furthermore, the remedies are not simply diluted but shaken at each stage of the dilution process. Hahnemann created this technique when he found that extreme levels of dilution would eradicate the side effects but not stop the effectiveness of a remedy. His new method (succussion) involved shaking with an impact rather than simply mixing the substance after each dilution and it is believed that this action releases the strength or energy of the 'potentised' remedy. Although no hard and fast explanation has yet been given, it cannot be denied that a considerable body of powerful anecdotal evidence has shown that homeopathic medicine emphatically does work. Countries that have a recognised and well-established track record with this therapy include India, France, Germany, Italy, Great Britain, South America and the United States.

differentiating between acute and chronic conditions

This book will give you all the information you need to know about treating all those minor health problems that are part and parcel of everyday life. All these will fall into the category of 'acute' conditions and will respond very well to home prescribing, which will be able to alleviate pain, dramatically shorten the duration of the illness and protect against further complications.

Acute conditions are those that have a specific, limited time span and that will, given appropriate support such as rest and recuperation, clear up of their own accord. They involve three clear-cut stages: the incubation period, when there may be no symptoms of the illness; the acute phase, when the symptoms are very recognisable; and the convalescent stage, when the patient begins to feel better. However, a few acute illnesses, such as pneumonia and meningitis, can be extremely serious and obviously fall outside the remit of a general acute condition as they require professional emergency treatment and management.

Chronic conditions are more deep-seated than acute diseases and do not clear up, however much time and appropriate support is made available. Instead, chronic problems are subject to flare-ups of symptoms at intermittent intervals which may or may not become more severe with the passage of time. Chronic conditions, like arthritis, high blood pressure, asthma and migraines, are best managed by professional homeopaths rather than home prescribing.

how homeopathy relates to conventional medicine

Homeopathy is an extremely practical and flexible form of therapy that can be applied to an impressively wide range of conditions, from first aid to acute or chronic problems. It therefore has the potential to be used both as a complete system of treatment in itself as well as in a support role with conventional medicine.

For example, homeopaths are regularly called on to treat babies and children who are suffering from infantile eczema. Conventional medical treatment usually involves the prescription of steroid creams that can have the negative side effect of thinning young and delicate skin. This is often a major concern to parents and therefore the homeopathic alternative provides a genuinely practical solution. The remedy Petroleum may take slightly longer to relieve inflammation and itching, but the results are impressive and far longer lasting than the temporary 'band aid' effect of steroid ointments. Indeed, there are many circumstances where homeopathy can provide a very valid alternative and especially with current concerns about the over-use of antibiotics leading to the development of superbugs, and over-reliance on pain killers leading to rebound headaches and even addiction.

Homeopathy also has great scope when used to support or 'complement' conventional medicine. The remedies are extremely dilute and therefore there is no danger of a harmful interaction between a remedy and a course of conventional drugs. Even if you are already taking an antibiotic, you can still gain some benefit from the additional use of homeopathy. For example, remedies such as Hepar sulph and Pulsatilla are good at breaking down and expelling mucus discharges and can therefore speed up the rate at which the infection is dealt with.

In my opinion, this form of integrated medical support provides the best of both worlds as it prioritises a holistic form of treatment but keeps more aggressive measures in reserve for situations that demand a more vigorous or heroic approach. It is the model that I have used for this book and therefore in each section, where appropriate, you will find pointers that suggest when you might need to consult your doctor.

how homeopathy is related to other complementary therapies

Generally speaking, homeopathy is compatible with most other non-conventional therapies such as Western medical herbalism, nutritional therapy and aromatherapy (although care needs to be taken with some specific essential oils that are thought to interfere with the medicinal action of homeopathic remedies). If you are receiving on-going treatment from a homeopathic practitioner do tell them about any other therapies you are using or considering using. They may want you to postpone any additional treatment until they have had a chance to evaluate your response to the homeopathic remedy they are prescribing; it's important to know what's doing what as otherwise it's difficult to work out which response relates to which measure. In this book, I have tried to keep things simple by indicating where extra help, in the form of herbal, nutritional or aromatherapy support, is appropriate. And in all these circumstances, you can take it for granted that it will be completely compatible with homeopathic home prescribing.

how to set about getting the basic information

Homeopathy lays a huge emphasis on tailoring treatment to every individual situation and is therefore in contrast to conventional medicine, which depends on a set of standard responses for specific conditions: decongestants for sinus problems and catarrh, antibiotics for bacterial infections, anti-fungal preparations for athlete's foot, and laxatives for constipation, etc. In contrast, homeopathic medicines are not prescribed for the condition but for the person who is experiencing symptoms of the condition. These symptoms are unique to that person. The common cold, for example, can affect half a dozen people suffering from the same virus in a different way. The most important thing to bear in mind is that you need to get to the essence of how feeling ill affects each person differently and how this goes beyond the physical complaints to include emotional and mental strains.

Effective homeopathic treatment depends on obtaining from the patient as complete and detailed a 'symptom picture' as possible, as this tells the homeopath what happens to them when they fall ill and how this differs from their normal state of health. It is important to gather as much information as possible; simply knowing that your child has a headache is not enough. There is no such thing as a single, straightforward, homeopathic headache remedy because there are many variations common to this complaint. One headache might be characterised by a throbbing pain in the temples that feels better for lying down in a dark room, while another might be a dull ache that requires gentle exercise in the fresh air. Always look for this kind of differentiating characteristic as it is these that will lead you to a well-chosen remedy. When you are assessing a symptom picture always write down your observations, together with the remedy that you prescribe as this will be a useful record to keep track of your family's health and remind you of a particularly effective remedy for a recurring complaint.

When taking down a symptom picture, it helps to know the kind of questions you need to ask. Write the answers down in a list format with bullet points as this will then allow you to prioritise the significant symptoms that will lead you to the correct remedy.

- **How long has the problem been around?**
- **Were there any triggering factors e.g. a shock, chill or major change in routine?**
- **Where is the problem located?**
- **Is there any pain, and, if so, what makes it better or worse, and what is the nature of the sensation (sharp, constant, intermittent, throbbing, etc)?**
- **Have there been any emotional reactions to not feeling well such as uncharacteristic tearfulness in someone who is normally very even-tempered, or anxiety in someone who is very calm as a rule?**
- **Has this sort of thing happened before?**
- **What generally makes someone feel better or worse since feeling ill? E.g. Do you feel better for warmth or cold, first thing in the morning, in the middle of the day, or late at night?**
- **Have there been any changes in body temperature such as feeling unusually hot or chilly?**

prioritising self-help

When you have taken down the case, go through the list of symptoms and draw three lines under those symptoms that feel especially intense or severe. Then do the same for anything that falls under the category of 'strange, rare and peculiar', such as nausea that's better for eating, a dry mouth without thirst, or a sense of chill that feels worse for exposure to heat. Also give three lines to any recent precipitating factor, such as physical or emotional trauma, becoming chilled, or being exposed to an unusual amount of stress. These symptoms should be grouped under the heading of 'typical features'.

Next, use two lines to identify more low-grade, emotional or general symptoms that, while not especially severe, still stand for any change from what is normal. These would include symptoms like physical, mental or emotional restlessness in someone who's normally calm and laid back, or a gregarious and sociable person wanting to be completely alone. These go under the heading of 'general symptoms'.

Don't worry too much at the moment about the distinction between these two groups of features as there is bound to be some degree of overlap between them. In fact, once you become familiar with using the homeopathic tables you will see that these distinctions are merely a guide and don't need to be applied too rigidly in order to find the appropriate homeopathic remedy.

The symptoms that are left are the ones that should be given one line. These are any features that make the patient feel generally better or worse, or factors that may ease or aggravate individual symptoms. For instance, a headache may feel better for contact with fresh, cool air, while the person may experience a general need to wrap up warmly. These go under headings of 'worse from' or 'better for'.

N.B. It helps to bear in mind that the information you are looking for must signify any change from that which is normal for the patient. For instance, if someone feels very cold when ill but is actually quite a chilly person anyway then this is not of special importance. However, a change from feeling constantly cold to suddenly hot and feverish, since being unwell, is worth noting.

choosing the appropriate dose

The most common homeopathic dosages to be bought from high street outlets, such as pharmacies or health food shops, are the 6c and 30c kinds and these are appropriate for sorting out any acute problem in the context of home prescribing. Any higher potencies can be obtained from specialist pharmacies but these are safest in the hands of trained homeopathic therapists rather than raw beginners. Indeed, it is important to take care with the higher potencies in order to avoid over-stimulating and possibly aggravating the symptoms. This can happen if a high potency remedy is repeated too frequently and over too long a period of time and therefore, in this context, experience is essential.

The 'c' in a description of a remedy stands for the centessimal scale and tells you that one drop of the mother tincture has been added to ninety-nine drops of diluted alcohol and shaken in order to render the starting potency of 1c. This process is then repeated, adding one drop of this potency to another ninety-nine drops of the dilutant before shaking again and repeating the process to create remedies on an ascending scale of 2c, 3c and so on. There is also a decimal scale (labelled with an 'x') that works on the same principle, the only difference being that one drop of the mother tincture is added to nine drops of alcohol or distilled water, and shaken in order to render the starting potency of 1x etc. Once you are confident that your choice of homeopathic remedy fits the symptom picture of the patient, you can follow the general guidelines as to what dose to take and how often:

- If the problem is mild in nature, of recent onset (within the last few hours or a maximum of twenty four), and is not causing undue emotional distress to the patient, a 6c potency is an appropriate dose to start with.
- If the problem is more intense and severe in nature, has developed slowly and insidiously over three or four days, and is making the patient emotional, anxious or upset, a 30c potency is appropriate.
- Don't worry if you feel that a 30c would be ideal but all you have in your homeopathic first aid kit is the appropriate remedy in a 6c, as it will still be effective if you up the 6c dose to four times a day. The most essential thing is a well-chosen remedy, as no amount of dosing with an incorrect match will do any good whatsoever. When prescribing is inaccurate, nothing much is likely to happen and if it is fairly close, but not quite right, there will be partial improvement but not enough to resolve the situation satisfactorily.

how often to give the selected remedy

- Problems that are low-grade in nature and of recent onset should respond well to one 6c tablet given every two hours for a maximum of three doses in 24 hours. If marked improvement sets in after the first dose, watch and wait, since this is a sign that the remedy is working well and, provided the improvement continues to hold, you will not need to give another dose.
- If there is only a very slight improvement after the first dose, give a second or if need be a third two hours later in the expectation that they will finish the job.
- Should you find the improvement has held well for a day but the following morning the same symptoms are back, repeat the same treatment regime.
- More intense situations that involve more severe symptoms (this can refer as much to the degree of pain experienced, as to the amount of mucus congestion, or the level of emotional distress) will require a 30c potency given every three hours, again up to a maximum of three doses a day. The same principles apply as above: once improvement has set in it's time to stop giving the remedy.

how long should I expect to go on giving a remedy?

Once again, this is dependent on the individual situation but the following guidelines should cover most eventualities:

- Most acute, minor problems should be resolved within two to three days. If no improvement is forthcoming within this time scale, you need to be considering a change of remedy. A visit to the doctor would be indicated for a cough that appears to have turned into a chest infection with yellow or green mucus being produced, or any sensation of pain in the chest. Likewise with a cold that has turned into a sinus or ear infection.
- More low-grade, insidious problems should be considerably improved within three to four days. If not, another course of action needs to be considered such as a change of remedy or introducing nutritional supplements or herbal medicines, like Echinacea and/or vitamin C for recurrent head colds, or vitamin C for minor skin break outs.
- If you suspect a situation is moving outside your remit, always seek a professional opinion. Depending on the situation, this could come from your local pharmacist, NHS helpline, or complementary practitioner.

possible reactions after giving a remedy

- The ideal response is steady improvement in all symptoms that continues under its own steam from the point of taking the initial dose. This is proof of a very well-chosen remedy. If you repeat the remedy after two hours, you should expect to see improvements within minutes, or a maximum of an hour.
- Symptoms remain much the same after an hour or so but the patient feels decidedly better in themselves. This is a positive response to a well-chosen remedy as it suggests that curative action is in motion and, within an hour or two, the symptoms will begin to ease. In this situation, only repeat your selected remedy if symptoms reappear at a later stage.
- Improvement of symptoms here and there but no major change for the better. This would suggest that the remedy was only partially appropriate so you need to assess the patient's symptoms again and consult the appropriate remedy table in order to see if another choice fits the symptom picture more accurately.
- Initial positive reaction to two or three doses of a 6c potency but when a relapse occurs, the symptoms don't respond at all. If the symptoms remain unchanged it's time to increase the dose to 30c, following the instructions suggested above.
- If the symptoms change after giving a well-indicated remedy, you need to go back to the

remedy table in order to find a new symptom fit. A good example is when a cold starts off with scanty, clear nasal discharge but then changes to produce a more profuse yellowish-green mucus as the cold goes through its stages. This is obviously quite normal but you must adjust the remedy to fit the new symptoms if you want improvement to continue.

• Sometimes there can be a brief intensification of symptoms if you give too high a potency of the most appropriate remedy. This is a good sign, confirming your choice of remedy, but you should stop taking the remedy in order to prevent prolonged aggravation of your symptoms.

• No improvement at all, even after repeating the remedy for the maximum of 48 hours, would suggest that an inappropriate remedy has been selected, or that the required potency is outside the realm of a home-prescribing situation. If this happens, and you can find no other appropriate remedy in the remedy tables, seek professional medical advice.

a sample case

Now you know the theory, this sample case of a bad hangover should guide you easily through the acute prescribing process.

Kate's complaint is a simple case of queasiness as a result of too many late nights out. Normally someone blessed with a cast-iron constitution (regularly working digestion etc.) she is appalled to wake up, after a night of particularly heavy drinking, feeling awful. The most noticeable symptoms are absolutely no appetite on waking with a nasty queasy sensation and a strong urge to empty the bowel but a feeling that any movement is incomplete. In addition, she has a classic hangover-type headache that feels really heavy at the back of the neck. Feeling generally very fragile, Kate feels even more sick at the thought of a restorative cup of coffee, the smell of cigarette smoke or even the slightest bite of food and just wants to crawl back into bed and go to sleep. The main symptoms to be taken from here are as follows:

• Too many late nights and too much alcohol are the precipitating factors or 'triggers' and therefore these are underlined three times, as well as the queasiness and the headache, which are severe and therefore typical symptoms

• The constipation is also important as this is a change from Kate's normal digestive state, and can we given two or three lines, depending on the degree of distress it is causing. Kate's lack of appetite is a general symptom and should therefore get two lines

• Worse from eating and drinking coffee and better for sound sleep and bed will get one underline because they are to be expected and can be grouped under 'worse from', or 'better for'

Now the basic list of symptoms has been prioritised, you can match the information to the appropriate homeopathic table on page 59.

selecting the appropriate homeopathic remedy with the quick-reference remedy tables

Kate's match with the remedy tables is going to be quite easy to find because the cause of her problem and the nature of the symptoms are very clear cut. This, unfortunately, will not always be the case as sometimes the situation appears more diffuse, such as with flu-like symptoms that develop insidiously over a few days without any obvious cause, or generally stress-related gastric upsets. However, there is no need to panic if you can't get the information you have gathered to fit exactly with the information in the tables. All you need is enough of an approximation to make the correct remedy choice.

With Kate's case, if you turn to the homeopathic table in the hangover section on page 59, you can see that you have a selection of three remedies to choose from: Nux vomica, Bryonia and Coffea. Kate's hangover could feasibly fit into all the three 'Type' columns as it could have been exacerbated both by the stress of too many late nights and by low-grade dehydration, which often accompanies even small amounts of alcohol consumption. We know from our notes that Kate really can't face the idea of coffee so it is impossible to rule out any of the remedies at this stage. However, when you look at the more detailed symptom picture it becomes far easier to differentiate between the remedies, as it is only the Nux vomica that lists both the severe headache on waking lodged at the back of the head, the nausea and the constipation with a strong urge to empty the bowel. Already you can be pretty sure you're on the right track, but you can then confirm you choice of remedy with a glance at the 'worse from' and 'better for' columns. Sure enough, Kate's specific aversion to coffee and cigarettes make their appearance, plus her need to curl up and go to sleep. At this point the remedy Nux vomica is a really sound choice.

cross-checking with the materia medica to confirm the choice of remedy

Returning one last time to Kate and her hangover you can confirm your choice of remedy by consulting the Materia Medica on page 243. This provides a quick-reference guide to the essential features of almost all the homeopathic remedies listed throughout this book. The information given in the tables provides you with a snapshot of a remedy that will often be sufficient to help you prescribe and yet, as you build up confidence it is worth cross-checking with the Materia Medica as it gives a full portrait of all the common remedies and will enable you to gain absolute confirmation.

The Materia Medica is especially valuable where you may be hovering between two remedies and not quite sure which way to go. Having a more detailed picture should make it obvious which one is going to be more suitable, even if it means you have to go back and get more information from the patient before making your final choice.

a note for beginners

If you are a true novice to homeopathic prescribing and all of this feels like quite a culture shock, start with the first aid section in Chapter Two. The beauty of starting here is that choosing remedies for simple first-aid problems is just about as close as you are ever going to come to routine prescribing in homeopathy. It is therefore a good way of getting a practical feel for the remedies and building up your confidence so that you can naturally progress to tailoring the remedies to the individual in later chapters.

In many first-aid situations, Arnica is the remedy that is best indicated as it is excellent for helping with the symptoms of psychological shock that accompany every small accident, while also encouraging the damaged tissues to reabsorb blood. Arnica eases pain, heals bruises speedily and encourages tenderness and swelling to go down impressively quickly. Furthermore, as you won't need to agonise over making the correct remedy choice, you can concentrate instead on getting the practical feel of how often a remedy needs to be repeated. If a particular remedy comes up time and time again, it's a good way of learning how a single homeopathic remedy can be used to treat many diverse conditions. Phosphorus, for example, can be used effectively at different times for nosebleeds, coughs, sinus infections and acute anxiety, provided the symptoms fit.

Working with first aid cases will also help you understand how to use homeopathy side by side with other complementary treatments which may include herbal creams and tinctures, or aromatherapy essential oils. For example, after a minor accident you can apply Arnica cream (a herbal product) topically to the bruises, take it in tablet form to help speed up the internal healing process and also sip a weak dilution of Rescue remedy (flower essence remedy) to ease a minor case of shock.

guidelines for taking homeopathic remedies

All the references to homeopathic remedies in the tables throughout the book will refer to medicines that are taken orally in tablet form, unless otherwise specified. Additional forms of medicinal support, such as aromatherapy oils, herbal tinctures and creams or ointments will be listed separately under the 'Practical Self-Help' sections.

• In theory, homeopathic remedies can be obtained in a wide variety of forms including tablets, powders, granules and pillules (which are round sucrose globules that may be soft or hard). However, for the purposes of home prescribing, you will be dealing with pharmacy-bought tablets that are made from a sucrose lactose (milk sugar) base to which the remedy has been added. (If you happen to be lactose intolerant, remedies are available as solutions which you drop directly onto the tongue.)

• The most important thing to know at the outset is that you only select and take one homeopathic remedy at a time. In other words, if you find a partial fit for your symptoms, don't combine this with a handful of others in the hope that something positive will happen. Instead, try to find the single remedy that covers the essential aspects of the symptoms as closely as possible. The better the match, the more impressive and lasting the results are likely to be.

• Once you have selected your remedy, gently shake one tablet into the cap of the bottle before tipping it into your mouth. Some homeopathic remedies come in smart click packs that allow you to decant one tablet at a time into the cap of the container. This means that you can place the tablet in your mouth without touching it with your fingers, therefore avoiding the risk of contamination. This is important as remedies can easily become less medicinally active as a result of overhandling.

• Because homeopathic remedies are understood to begin working as soon as they make contact with the mucus membranes in the mouth, avoid drinking or chewing on any strong flavours before, or immediately after taking the remedy. Steer clear of peppermints, strong coffee or tea, cigarettes and toothpaste for at least thirty minutes before or after taking a remedy.

• If the tablet has a sufficiently soft milk sugar base it can be left to dissolve in the mouth. However, the hard varieties will need to be chewed, or they will sit for hours before eventually melting. Thankfully the taste is not at all unpleasant; just mildly sweet from the milk sugar base.

• In order to give your homeopathic remedies the best chance of a long shelf life it is helpful to keep the bottle caps well screwed on and to avoid prolonged exposure to sunlight. I would also recommend that you store them away from aromatic perfumes such as peppermint, eucalyptus and other essential oils, as strong smells of any kind can make the pills lose their potency.

• If you absent-mindedly take more than one tablet at a time (this has happened to more than one of my patients!), don't panic. Unlike using conventional medicines where the size of the dose is of great importance, the frequency with which homeopathic medicines are given is considered to be far more significant. For instance, if six tablets are taken at the same time, this constitutes a single dose. But if one of these tablets was taken at hourly intervals until they were all used up, then that would constitute six doses and would be regarded as having a cumulative effect.

putting together a homeopathic first-aid kit

You can buy ready-made homeopathic kits from a pharmacy and these are often good value for money. However, if you decide to put together one of your own, you can tailor the contents to your family's requirements. You won't need to buy everything all at once, just start with a small number of the first-aid remedies that are most appropriate for your needs, and then gradually add to the selection as the opportunity arises. In addition to your basic range of homeopathic remedies in tablet form you will also find it useful to have a small range of herbal creams and tinctures in your kit, as well as a small selection of essential oils. I have listed everything that is appropriate in the breakdown of each kit's contents on page 22.

where and how to purchase these items

All the products mentioned below are easily obtained by shopping at your local health food shop and/or high street pharmacy and, if anything should turn out to be unusually elusive, I have provided a list of addresses on page 282 that will point you in the direction of specialist outlets. Here, staff will be trained to answer any queries you may have over the phone and remedies can be sent out by mail order service. Most homeopathic pharmacies will also stock extra complementary medical products such as herbal tinctures, ointments and creams.

additional help and support

If you would like to get some formal training in homeopathic therapy, you can attend a basic first aid and home prescribing course that generally run for approximately six weeks at a time. These are aimed at giving the average interested member of the public a basic grounding in home prescribing and are an excellent way of gaining confidence for the beginner. All courses are led by a trained practitioner and are very interactive which means you can answer all the queries that accompany the practical application of homeopathy.

ringing the changes: selecting the contents of a starter kit

The following are lists of the most basic remedies that you will need, and which you can add to over time in order to build up indispensable, personalised kits.

FUNDAMENTAL HOMEOPATHIC REMEDIES

Aconite 6c – for colds and fevers after exposure to dry, cold winds, panic and anxiety

Arnica 6c – for bruises, muscle strain and shock from minor accidents

Belladonna 6c – for sunburn and the early stages of sore throats

Gelsemium 6c – for flu-like symptoms, anticipatory anxiety and headaches

Nux vomica 6c – for hangovers, constipation and headaches from lack of sleep and stress

Pulsatilla 6c – for established colds, coughs, earaches and swollen glands

Calendula tincture (this is a concentrated liquid that needs to be diluted before use)

Calendula cream – both promote the healing of damaged tissue by speeding up the production of healthy skin tissue and acting as a natural antiseptic

Lavender essential oil – Soothing to the skin; helps ease minor burns; also sleep-inducing and relaxing

ACCIDENT AND EMERGENCY KIT

Arnica 6c – for bruises, muscle strain and shock from minor accidents

Apis 6c – for bites, stings and fluid retention

Bryonia 6c – for headaches, dry, tickly coughs, sprains and strains

Cantharis 6c – for cystitis and minor burns

Carbo veg 6c – for fainting and gastric upsets

Ledum 6c – for bites, stings, strains, sprains and black eyes

Rhus tox 6c – for itchy skin, sprains and strains

Symphytum 6c – for fractures and black eyes

Urtica urens 6c – for stings, minor burns, scalds and sunburn

Calendula tincture – promotes the healing of damaged tissue

Hypericum tinctures – soothes any injury to areas rich in nerves

Urtica urens tincture – eases discomfort from bites and minor burns

Eucalyptus essential oil – clears congestion

Geranium essential oil – uplifting and calming

Lavender essential oil – soothing to the skin; helps ease minor burns; also sleep-inducing and relaxing

Tea tree essential oil – antibacterial

COMPREHENSIVE KIT

This will give you a flexible range of remedies that should deal with most of the acute problems that may occur in your family:

Aconite 6c – for colds and fevers after exposure to dry, cold winds, panic and anxiety

Arnica 6c – for bruises, muscle strain and shock from minor accidents

Arsenicum album 6c – for gastric upsets, anxiety, dry coughs and colds

Belladonna 6c – for sunburn and the early stages of sore throats

Bryonia 6c – for headaches, dry, tickly coughs, sprains and strains

Carbo veg 6c – for fainting and gastric upsets

Chamomilla 6c – for teething pains, stomach cramps and baby colic

Gelsemium 6c – for flu-like symptoms, anticipatory anxiety and headaches

Ignatia 6c – for grief, stomach upsets and stress-related problems

Lycopodium 6c – for anticipatory anxiety, gastric upsets and stress-related problems

Nux vomica 6c – for hangovers, constipation and headaches from lack of sleep and stress

Phosphorus 6c – for sinus pain and congestion, coughs, diarrhoea and anxiety

Pulsatilla 6c – for the established stage of colds, coughs, earaches and swollen glands

Calendula tincture and cream – both promote the healing of damaged tissue by speeding up the production of healthy skin tissue and acting as a natural antiseptic

Aloe vera gel – soothing, anti-inflammatory

Arnica cream – relieves pain and swelling of bruises, muscle aching and tenderness

Echinacea elixir or tincture – (this is a liquid that can be taken orally) helps immune system functioning

Eucalyptus essential oil – clears congestion

Lavender essential oil – soothing to the skin, helps ease minor burns, also sleep-inducing and relaxing

Rescue remedy – (to be taken orally in spray form or diluted in a glass of water) eases trauma

Slippery elm tablets or powder – soothes digestion

Tea tree essential oil – antibacterial

MOTHER AND BABY KIT

Arnica 6c – for bruises, muscle strain and shock from minor accidents
Bryonia 6c – for mastitis and irritability
Chamonilla 6c – for teething pains, stomach cramps and baby colic
Colocynthis 6c – for soothing stomach cramps and colic
Ferrum phos 6c – for the early stage of infection e.g. earaches and sore throats
Kreosotum 6c – for thrush and teething pains
Mag phos 6c – for teething, colic, wind and neuralgic pain
Calendula tincture and cream – both promote the healing of damaged tissue by speeding up the production of healthy skin tissue and acting as a natural antiseptic
Chamomile essential oil - relaxing
Lavender essential oil – soothing to the skin, helps ease minor burns, also sleep-inducing and relaxing
Rescue remedy – eases trauma

CHILDREN'S KIT

Aconite 6c – for colds and fevers after exposure to dry, cold winds, panic and anxiety
Arnica 6c – for bruises, muscle strain and shock from minor accidents
Bellladonna 6c – for sunburn and the early stages of sore throats
Calc carb 6c – for chapped skin, cradle cap, nappy rash and slow, painful teething
Chamomilla 6c – for teething pains, stomach cramps and baby colic
Ignatia 6c – for grief, stomach upsets and stress-related problems
Nux vomica 6c – for constipation and headaches from lack of sleep and stress
Phosphorus 6c – for sinus pain and congestion, coughs, diarrhoea and anxiety
Pulsatilla 6c – for the established stage of colds, coughs, earaches and swollen glands
Arnica cream – relieves pain and swelling of bruises, muscle aching and tenderness
Calendula cream –promotes the healing of damaged tissue by speeding up the production of healthy skin tissue and acting as a natural antiseptic

CAUTION!
signs that suggest that medical advice is needed

• Should you have an instinct that the problem is deteriorating, always err on the side of caution and get a medical opinion. For minor skin conditions that are proving stubborn to clear up, you can wait until you get an appointment at your doctor's surgery. However, more pressing, acute situations, and especially those that involve babies, young children and the elderly, will require a fast medical response. Situations of this kind are described in the Caution! sections under each condition heading.

• When evaluating a deteriorating condition, you should be as concerned with how the patient feels in themselves, as you are about the specific look and nature of the individual symptoms. So, even if a headache, sore throat, or cough seem to be much the same in nature but the patient feels generally much more unwell, this should be taken as a sign that things are getting worse.

• If it becomes necessary to keep up a long term, low potency dose of a remedy in order to maintain an improvement, it is a sign that the situation has moved into the sphere of a chronic condition and, as such, it will be helpful to consult an experienced homeopathic practitioner. Always bear in mind that low potency homeopathic remedies are only intended to be taken in the very short-term as a way of kick-starting a curative response. They are not designed to be taken as more permanent support.

CAUTION!
signs that suggest that emergency medical help is needed

- Any sign of disorientation, confusion, and/or drowsiness.
- Rapidly-rising temperature that reaches 103°F or 39–40°C.
- Muscle stiffness and aching that's combined with a severe headache and light sensitivity.
- Loss of consciousness.
- Severe or long-lasting loss of body fluids through vomiting, diarrhoea or blood loss.
- Suspicion of infection due to a high temperature, inflammation and formation of pus.
- Severe illness in the very young or the very elderly.

finding a homeopathic practitioner

Throughout the book I have recommended where it might be appropriate to consult an experienced homeopathic practitioner. Chronic conditions that respond well to deep-acting treatment that's aimed at getting the whole system into optimum balance (known as constitutional prescribing) include migraines, irritable bowel syndrome, mild to moderate depression and anxiety, eczema, asthma and psoriasis to name just a few.

Generally speaking, the best way of finding a reliable therapist is through an enthusiastic recommendation from someone whose opinion you know you can trust. In the absence of this personal network, you can obtain a register of qualified homeopaths from the Society of Homeopaths and this will contain a list of qualified practitioners who have satisfied the stringent criteria for being entered onto the Society's register. This includes having graduated through an approved training and having satisfied the requirements of providing evidence of reflective practice and being observed on a site visit. This constitutes an assessment of the practitioner's general sense of professionalism, as well as their academic grasp of their subject and, most significantly of all, their interaction and rapport with their patients. Those practitioners who are successfully registered use the initials RS Hom along with any other qualifications after their name.

Alternatively, if you feel you would prefer to consult a homeopathic practitioner who is also qualified in conventional medicine, you should contact the British Homeopathic Association who will be able to supply you with a list of practitioners. These will use the letters MF Hom after their name.

2 | homeopathy and first aid

This is the place to start for anyone new to homeopathic prescribing as acute first-aid conditions, such as cuts, scrapes and bruises, are more straightforward and routine than coughs, colds and stomach upsets, which tend to have quite individualised symptoms. Once you have gained confidence by getting good results with first-aid situations, you will then be ready to move on to the slightly more challenging prescribing in the later chapters of this book.

It helps right at the outset to be aware that you can use homeopathy safely with any practical first-aid measures. In fact, it's positively helpful to do so, as when remedies work effectively, it speeds up the process of general recovery in double-quick time. For example if you apply a cold compress or ice pack to a bad bruise (provided the skin has not been broken) and also take Arnica tablets internally, then both these strategies will assist the body to do the same thing, which is taking down the swelling and easing the localised pain and tenderness. However, the Arnica is also able to provide the added therapeutic advantage of encouraging the traumatised tissues to re-absorb blood.

The beauty of homeopathic prescribing at this level is that you can reasonably expect to see positive results within a very short period of time. In cases of minor bruises, cuts and grazes, you should see signs of efficient healing within two or three days. And if you are worried about getting out of your depth, just look at the advice listed in the 'Caution!' sections for these will give you a clear indication of when you need to get a professional assessment or, in some cases, emergency medical help.

minor bruises

Bruising is most likely to occur as part and parcel of a fall or minor mishap, such as stubbing your toe or accidentally hammering your finger during some routine DIY. However a serious accident can result in quite severe internal bruising and this would fall outside the remit of home prescribing and demand urgent, professional medical attention. Common symptoms of mild bruising can include any of the following:

- **Pain and tenderness at the site of the blow or injury**
- **Swelling of the injured area**
- **Localised, progressive discolouration of the skin that changes from red to purple and eventually to a rather lurid bluish-greeny-yellow in the last stages of healing**

practical self-help

❧ As long as the skin around the bruise hasn't been broken, apply an ice pack to ease pain and reduce inflammation.

❧ Bruises, where the skin hasn't been cut or grazed, can be greatly soothed by an application of Arnica cream. This reduces any pain and tenderness and also encourages the traumatised tissue to reabsorb blood, thereby speeding up the healing process.

❧ If a limb has been badly bruised, keep it moving as much as possible in order to keep the blood circulating.

❧ Witch hazel has a very soothing, cooling effect on bruised skin. However, it is highly astringent and therefore may not be suitable for anyone with very sensitive skin.

CAUTION!

IF ANY OF THE FOLLOWING OCCUR, GET SWIFT MEDICAL ASSISTANCE:

- **A serious fall or major accident that has resulted in the casualty feeling drowsy or confused**
- **Any injury to the head**
- **Bruising of the eye socket**
- **In addition, get your doctor's opinion if you notice that the skin is repeatedly bruising for no reason, or if bruises take longer than a few days to heal – ideally, even a nasty bruise shouldn't take longer than this to show signs of recovery**

TYPE OF BRUISE	GENERAL SYMPTOMS	WORSE FROM	BETTER FOR	REMEDY NAME
Simple bruises from any minor trauma or accident	- Arnica is one of the few remedies that can be given routinely for any minor injury – not only does it help bruises heal, but it also eases any slight shock symptoms that may accompany a minor accident	- Motion - Making any effort - Touch	- Resting	**Arnica**
Deep bruising	- This remedy follows Arnica very well and can resolve well-established, deep-seated bruising - It is especially well indicated after surgery	- Touch - Hot bathing	- Cool bathing - Moving about	**Bellis perennis**
Bruising to the eye socket	- Once a conventional medical opinion has been obtained, this remedy can be invaluable in healing bruising around the eye that has happened as a result of contact with a blunt object (e.g. a tennis ball)	- Touch		**Symphytum**
Black eyes that feel cold and numb	- Lots of swelling, tenderness and sensitivity around the affected area - Pains are likely to feel stabbing or tearing in nature	- Warmth - Moving about	- Contact with cool, fresh air - Cool bathing - Rest	**Ledum**
Bruises that affect areas of the body where the skin is thin (e.g. the shins)	- This remedy is especially well indicated where the periosteum (the sensitive, fibrous connective tissue that is wrapped around the bones) has been bruised as this can cause pain that remains long after superficial bruising has healed	- Walking - Touch - Rest - Lying on the bruised part	- Staying indoors - Warmth	**Ruta**

cuts, grazes and wounds

Minor kitchen accidents and DIY mishaps tend to be the most common causes of minor abrasions in adults but for children, cuts, scrapes and bruises are an inevitable part of playtime and so it helps to have something on hand to make it all better. The self-help treatments outlined below will encourage minor, straightforward cuts and grazes to heal quickly, while easing discomfort and minimising the risk of infection.

practical self-help

❧ Bathe and clean the wound with a diluted tincture of Calendula. For optimal results one part tincture should be diluted in ten parts boiled, cooled water.

❧ Small puncture wounds should be cleaned and bathed with a similar dilution of Hypericum and Calendula tincture (1:1:10); the Calendula acts as a natural antiseptic while also encouraging the skin to heal and the Hypericum works as an additional pain reliever.

❧ Once the wound is thoroughly clean, pat dry before adding Calendula cream and covering with a sterile dressing. You can also add Calendula cream to the surface of the dressing to encourage swift healing.

CAUTION!

• Because Calendula is so effective at encouraging wounds to heal in double-quick time, always make sure that there's no residual debris left in a wound or graze before you apply the cream – the last thing you want is to seal in the infection at a deeper level

IF ANY OF THE FOLLOWING OCCUR, GET SWIFT MEDICAL ASSISTANCE:

• Wide and/or deep cuts that can't easily be held together by dressings, or large jagged cuts, especially when these have been sustained over a joint, such as the knee

• Any sign of numbness, tingling or weakness in the injured area

• Any indication that infection is beginning to develop. The most obvious signs include redness, heat, or pus formation around the injury. If red streaks begin to radiate from the wound, or if a high fever develops (39°C/102°F), get medical help at once

TYPE OF WOUND	GENERAL SYMPTOMS	WORSE FROM	BETTER FOR	REMEDY NAME
Minor cuts and grazes with mild shock	- A sense of being generally shaken up as a result of a minor fall or abrasion, especially if it's combined with some bruising	- Being fussed over - Touch - Moving	- Resting with the head lower than the body	**Arnica**
Wounds to nerve-dense areas, such as the hands or feet	- Pains are likely to feel intermittently sharp and shooting and may radiate away from the cut - The affected area feels sore and hypersensitive to touch	- Contact with cool air - Touch - Moving the injured area	- Keeping the affected area as still as possible	**Hypericum**
Puncture wounds that feel cool to the touch	- Pains in and around the wound are sharp and stabbing or tearing in nature - There is likely to be intense sensitivity to the pain	- Heat locally applied - At night - Movement	- Contact with cool air - Cool bathing and/or cool compresses locally applied - Rest	**Ledum**
Wounds that have a raised, rosy-pink look	- Pains are stinging and sharp in and around the wound - Localised puffiness around the cut	- Contact with warm air - Resting - Warm bathing	- Cool bathing - Gentle motion	**Apis**

homeopathy

sprains and strains

Sprains and strains often occur because of a sudden movement that injures the tendons of a joint, but can also be the result of repeated stressful movements that overtax a muscle or joint a little more each time until you start to feel the discomfort. Be especially careful when you take up a vigorous exercise regime after years of being a confirmed couch potato and always remember to limber up first. Common symptoms are likely to include:

- **Pain, inflammation and stiffness around the affected area**
- **Discomfort on moving the damaged part, especially at first**
- **Skin discolouration around the injured area**

practical self-help

FOR SPRAINS...

❧ If the skin hasn't been broken, apply an ice pack as soon as possible to reduce swelling and pain.

❧ After the ice pack, apply a cold compress of diluted Arnica tincture (once again, do not do this if the skin has been cut). Soak a clean cloth in the liquid (one part tincture to ten parts boiled, cooled water), wring out and then hold it against the injured area for as long as feels soothing.

❧ Bind the affected limb with a supportive crepe bandage and rest it for at least two days following the injury. If swelling is pronounced, keep it in a comfortably raised position as this encourages the swelling to drain away more efficiently.

practical self-help

FOR STRAINS...

❧ If a strained muscle feels more comfortable for being strapped up in a support bandage, make sure that it isn't too tight and obstructing circulation to the affected limb.

❧ As soon as the pain has eased, gently start moving the affected muscle or muscle groups to avoid losing strength and bulk as a result of extended lack of use – it's incredible how quickly immobile muscles become weak.

❧ Regular applications of Arnica cream to strained muscles can do an impressive amount to relieve discomfort and speed up recovery.

❧ Severe muscle strains are often initially eased by Arnica cream but then stop making good progress. For these cases, switch to Ruta ointment.

TYPE OF SPRAIN OR STRAIN	GENERAL SYMPTOMS	WORSE FROM	BETTER FOR	REMEDY NAME
Swelling, minor shock and pain following any injury	- Bruising, swelling and inflammation; tissues feel incredibly tender and sensitive to touch	- Motion - Touch	- Resting - Being left to get on with it and not being fussed over	**Arnica**
Later stages of strains/sprains that are eased by movement	- Once Arnica has stopped being effective, stiffness and tenderness is obviously aggravated when at rest - Emotionally low and depressed	- Initial movement - Prolonged movement - Chill	- Warm bathing - Gentle motion that doesn't overtax	**Rhus tox**
Later stages of strains/sprains that feel better for rest	- Lots of inflammation with a sense of heat and redness in the affected area - Feels much more comfortable for support that gives firm pressure	- Even the slightest motion - Getting up after sitting for a while - Light touch	- Firm pressure to the painful area - Keeping very still in one position	**Bryonia**
Repetitive strain injuries	- This remedy is most useful for injuries affecting the wrist, knee and ankle joints that result from long-term strain rather than a short, sharp injury	- Lying on the painful part - Touch - Cold and damp	- Warmth	**Ruta**
Sprains and strains that feel internally cold	- Although the affected area is hot and swollen, it feels cold to the touch - Getting warm increases the discomfort	- Warm bathing - Motion - Becoming heated	- Cool bathing - Coolness, locally applied - Draughts of cool air	**Ledum**

homeopathy

31

CAUTION!

- Call for medical help if a sprained joint remains unusable for 24 hours after the accident has happened, or if there are any obvious signs of distortion and/or marked disolouration or numbness

minor burns and scalds

Most minor burns happen in the kitchen from contact with extremely hot surfaces, such as ovens or electric hobs. However, they can also be caused by too much sun exposure or falling against central heating radiators that are on too high a setting. Minor scalds happen easily if you accidentally reach over a boiling kettle or saucepan, or spill a very hot drink, and excessively hot baths can also inflict nasty scalds so always check the water while it is running. Symptoms of low-grade burns and scalds are likely to include any combination of the following, in varying degrees of severity:

- **Stinging and burning skin**
- **Localised redness, heat and inflammation of the area that's been damaged**
- **Blisters form to protect the skin that needs to heal underneath. Because of their protective role, resist the temptation to burst a blister as otherwise infection can easily set in**

practical self-help

❧ Bathing the affected area in a cool solution of Urtica urens tincture feels beautifully soothing to stinging skin, while also encouraging healing to take place quickly and efficiently. For best results, dilute one part tincture to ten parts boiled, cooled water.

❧ If blisters have broken, use diluted Calendula tincture to discourage infection and speed up recovery. Dilute as suggested for Urtica urens tincture above.

❧ After bathing has calmed down the localised heat and inflammation, massage a soothing salve into the area to speed up recovery and reduce discomfort. Dilute ten drops of lavender essential oil in a teaspoonful of gel base or Urtica urens cream. However, if a blister has broken, Calendula cream or ointment is more suitable as its natural anti-bacterial properties discourage infection. (N.B. If you have sensitive skin, avoid the ointment due to its lanolin content.)

❧ Even the most undramatic minor accidents can still cause a shock and therefore a few drops of Rescue Remedy, either diluted in a small glass of water or placed directly under the tongue, can be very good for steadying the nerves.

TYPE OF BURN OR SCALD	GENERAL SYMPTOMS	WORSE FROM	BETTER FOR	REMEDY NAME
Minor burns with lots of stinging or burning without blistering	- First degree burns that look red and inflamed and feel either itchy or burning - A good tip for efficient healing is to take this remedy internally while also bathing the skin with the diluted tincture	- Touch		**Urtica urens**
After pains following burns or scalds	- Twinges of soreness and discomfort may remain after the skin has superficially healed	- Changes of temperature - Exposure to a draught or cold	- Resting - Being comfortably warm	**Causticum**
General minor shock symptoms	- Classic signs of shock after minor trauma include denial that anything is the matter and avoiding displays of concern or attention – if this happens, give Arnica first and then follow up with a specific burn/scald remedy	- Fuss and bother - Touch - Jarring	- Resting with the head lower than the body	**Arnica**

homeopathy

●

33

CAUTION!

IF ANY OF THE FOLLOWING OCCUR, GET SWIFT MEDICAL ASSISTANCE:

- **Severe burns or scalds that cover a skin surface area of more than 2.5 cm (1 inch) in diameter**
- **Burns sustained on the face, in the mouth, or over or around a joint**
- **Any signs of infection developing in, or around a burn or scald, e.g. persistent swelling, heat, redness and pus formation**

minor shock

When talking about shock it is important to clarify terms so that you know exactly what it is that you're dealing with, as the technical definition can be used to cover a significant range of emotions; from a brief reaction to a minor mishap to life-threatening symptoms that need the most urgent medical care. The self-help measures below are appropriate for minor, unsettling symptoms that are likely to resolve themselves in time, such as:

- **A sense of disorientation and anxiety**
- **Rapid pulse**
- **Uncharacteristic tearfulness**
- **Faintness and/or dizziness**

Severe shock, however, is a quite different animal and because of the severe nature of the condition, such as a major allergic reaction or an accident resulting in internal bleeding, symptoms tend to be equally dramatic and may include any of the following:

- **Rapidly-developing swelling and/or puffiness around the throat, lips and/or eyes**
- **Drowsiness and/or confusion**
- **Unconsciousness**
- **Difficult or irregular breathing patterns**
- **Collapse**
- **Skin that feels clammy to the touch and looks pale, possibly tinged with blue**
- **Nausea**

practical self-help

✽ It's almost always helpful to sit down and have a warm drink when in a state of shock and especially if faintness and disorientation are a problem. If a herbal blend like chamomile, lemon verbena or passiflora isn't easily available then Indian tea will do.

✽ Dilute a few drops of Rescue Remedy in a small glass of water and sip as often as needed in order to induce a feeling of calm.

✽ Putting a drop or two of lavender essential oil on a tissue and inhaling at frequent intervals can help the mild anxiety that often accompanies a slight shock.

TYPE OF SHOCK	GENERAL SYMPTOMS	WORSE FROM	BETTER FOR	REMEDY NAME
Basic shock reaction as a result of a minor accident or injury	- Shaken up, upset and generally wanting to get back to normal as quickly as possible	- Any fuss - Touch	- Resting quietly	**Arnica**
Emotional shock and panic from hearing bad news or seeing an accident	- Feelings of panic and fear may occur at the time of the traumatic incident or they may set in as a delayed reaction - Panicky, extremely restless or wobbly with sudden loss of strength	- Becoming chilled - Lots of noise or bright light - Touch	- Cool, fresh air that doesn't chill - Sound rest	**Aconite**
Feeling faint as a result of shock	- May pass out briefly as a response to shock, or feel as if about to collapse - Marked craving for cool air with a strong desire to be fanned - Skin looks pale and sweaty	- Overheated rooms - Tight clothes around the neck and waist	- Cool, fresh air that doesn't chill - Elevating the feet	**Carbo veg**
Emotional shock of bereavement	- Sighing and emotionally very changeable: moves very quickly from tears to laughter - Tense and nervous with disturbed sleep and a tendency to nightmares	- Fright - Being touched - Walking in the open air	- Being alone - Taking deep breaths - Small meals and snacks	**Ignatia**

homeopathy

●

3 5

CAUTION!

IF ANY OF THE CRITICAL SYMPTOMS DESCRIBED OPPOSITE SHOW SIGNS OF DEVELOPING, LOSE NO TIME IN GETTING EMERGENCY MEDICAL HELP. WHILE WAITING FOR PROFESSIONAL ASSISTANCE, IT HELPS TO DO THE FOLLOWING:

• **Loosen any tight clothing around the neck and waist**

• **If indoors, make sure that the surrounding temperature is neither too hot nor too cold**

recuperation after dental treatment

However sophisticated techniques of modern dentistry have undeniably become, it's still a fact that a lot of people avoid going for dental work if they possibly can, for fear of the treatment. Fortunately, the reality is often far less unpleasant and traumatic than the anticipation and 'catastrophising' that can cloud the run up to an appointment and so it is important that you don't let nerves stand in the way between you and a regular dentist check up. The following practical complementary steps can help dispel this psychological tension as well as speed up the healing process and ease any residual pain and discomfort.

practical self-help

❧ Rinsing the mouth with a solution of Calendula tincture after fillings, crown work or an extraction can do a great deal to help traumatised, bruised, or lacerated tissues heal in double-quick time. Dilute one part tincture in ten parts boiled, cooled water.

❧ If there is some residual sharp pain from the local anaesthetic injection at the site of the needle entry, a more effective mouthwash can be made up by diluting one part Hypericum tincture in ten parts boiled, cooled water.

❧ Mouth ulcers, often caused by the tissue being nicked slightly during treatment, can be encouraged to heal by using either of the mouthwashes mentioned above. Alternatively, dab the ulcer gently with a drop of tea tree essential oil on a cotton wool bud and then, after ten minutes, rinse the mouth out thoroughly with water.

❧ Jittery feelings that set in after coming home (often intensified by the adrenalin component in the local anaesthetic) can be eased by taking a few drops of Rescue Remedy diluted in a small glass of water.

CAUTION!

Never take Arnica after a tooth extraction as this remedy promotes the re-absorption of blood. This can lead to painful complications in the form of a dry socket that can take a very long time to heal

TYPE OF TRAUMA FROM DENTAL WORK	GENERAL SYMPTOMS	WORSE FROM	BETTER FOR	REMEDY NAME
General trauma and bruising to mouth (excluding extractions)	- Overall feeling of tenderness and soreness in the mouth that makes it very painful to chew	- Touch - Motion - After sleeping	- Resting with the head lower than the body	**Arnica**
Nerve pains following tooth extraction or pains at the site of a local anaesthetic injection	- Shooting pains around the area of dental work with more tenderness than would be expected from the size of the wound	- Jarring motion - Making a physical effort - Touch	- Tilting the head backwards	**Hypericum**
Deep, bruised pains after fillings not resolved by Arnica	- Residual aching after a deep filling or preparation work for crowns - General sense of restlessness because of persistent aching in the treated area	- Contact with cold - Stooping or bending forward - Lying down	- Warmth - Rubbing	**Ruta**
Pains caused by a dry tooth socket after extraction	- Great sensitivity to pain that feels squeezing, stinging or smarting - Pains following wisdom tooth extraction may feel especially excruciating around the area of the wound	- Cold drinks - Contact where the incision was made - During the night	- Warmth - Resting	**Staphysagria**

stings and insect bites

Most stings and insect bites are merely an irritant but they can also be quite painful and anyone who attracts the midges will be able to tell you how they can take the pleasure out of an otherwise enjoyable holiday. Furthermore, while the sting itself may not be harmful, anyone who is allergic must get emergency medical treatment in order to avoid anaphylactic shock as this very serious condition, if left untreated, can be fatal. Common symptoms include:

- **Signs of breathing difficulties, such as wheezing, gasping or obviously laboured breaths**
- **Extreme pallor and clamminess**
- **Collapse**
- **Shallow, rapid pulse**
- **Puffiness or noticeable swelling of the eyes, lips, throat, and/or face**

practical self-help

❧ Bathe inflamed, stinging, and/or itchy bites with a solution of Urtica urens tincture. Dilute one part tincture in ten parts boiled, cooled water and apply as often as feels soothing. This is particularly good for nettle stings.

❧ Bathe bee stings, once the sting has been carefully removed, with a solution of Calendula tincture, following the directions above.

❧ Place just one drop of lavender essential oil on the sensitive, inflamed skin and repeat at hourly intervals until the discomfort has subsided.

❧ If none of the above are readily available, ransack the kitchen cupboard. For wasp stings or flea bites make up a solution of vinegar or lemon juice and cold water, and for bee stings a weak solution of bicarbonate of soda and cold water.

❧ Rescue Remedy can do a great deal to calm the situation down if a degree of emotional shock accompanies the localised pain, especially with children or anyone who has a fear of wasps or bees. Dilute a few drops in a small glass of water and sip as often as necessary.

❧ If you know you attract insect bites like the plague and are travelling to an area where midges are known to thrive, make use of a natural insect repellant such as Pyrethrum spray (see stockists on page 282). Wear light nightclothes that provide cover for your arms and legs and don't wear anything too scented out of doors, as this can attract them.

CAUTION!

If there are any signs of extreme localised puffiness around the insect bite or sting that refuses to go down after a few hours, or if signs of infection develop, it's time to call on professional medical help

TYPE OF INSECT BITE OR STING	GENERAL SYMPTOMS	WORSE FROM	BETTER FOR	REMEDY NAME
Bee stings with pale pink, puffy swelling around the affected area	- The area around the sting looks raised and swollen - Stinging, burning pains that react very badly to heat in any form - This remedy also eases hives that can be triggered by a sting	- Any fuss - Touch	- Cool air - Cool bathing	**Apis**
Emotional shock or panic that follows being stung or bitten	- The affected area may look swollen and feel as though it's burning - The main problem is likely to be a hypersensitivity to pain – often intensified by feelings of fear and panic after the event	- Offers of help - Becoming chilled - Becoming overheated	- Rest	**Aconite**
Midge bites that are unbearably sensitive and/or itchy	- Discomfort from bites feels excruciatingly sharp and stinging; even the lightest contact from clothing is uncomfortable	- Touch of any kind	- Having a good initial scratch - Warmth	**Staphysagria**
Stings and insect bites of any kind that feel numb and cold to the touch	- Lots of localised redness and swelling with prickling pains - While the site of the bite or sting feels cold, it is made much less uncomfortable for contact with anything cool	- Becoming warm or warmth locally applied	- Uncovering - Cool air - Cool bathing	**Ledum**
Bee stings with localised burning around the affected area	- Stinging and itching around the sting - Hives may follow once the sting has healed - In contrast to Apis and Ledum, stings that are suited to this remedy feel worse for contact with cool air	- Bathing - Touch - Cool air		**Urtica urens**

homeopathy

●

39

sports injuries

While adopting a regular exercise regime is to be recommended for all the advantages it brings to your state of health and wellbeing, there are also, unfortunately, the aches and sprains that inevitably crop up at one time or another. Within this context, appropriate homeopathic prescribing, backed up with whatever conventional medical support is available (such as physiotherapy), can do a great deal to speed up the healing process of sports injuries.

achilles tendonitis

This is one of the most dreaded sports injuries due to the excruciating pain that sets in when the Achilles tendon (positioned just above the heel) becomes overstretched or partly ruptured. Unfortunately this injury can happen fairly readily as a result of a sudden jarring movement to the heel. As always, prevention is the best policy so....

- **Always warm up the muscles before a run, or beginning a workout in the gym – especially one that involves treadmill work or using a stationary cycle**
- **Avoid running on hard, inflexible surfaces or uneven ground as this causes constant jarring Choose resilient, grassy surfaces that put less strain on the heels, ankles, knees and hips**
- **Invest in good-quality running shoes that provide effective support and cushioning**
- **Take particular care if you set high fitness goals for yourself and always listen to your body**

practical self-help

❧ If you experience any pain in the heel, don't put it under strain for at least two weeks in order to avoid triggering a tendon spasm. Opt for non-weight-bearing forms of exercise, such as swimming, instead.

❧ Apply an ice pack or bag of frozen peas to the painful inflamed area for fifteen minutes at a time in order to reduce the pain and take down some of the swelling. However, do not apply a heavily frozen object directly to the skin as this can burn.

❧ Elevate the injured leg on a pillow or a cushion to encourage the swelling to go down.

❧ Massage the injured area daily with Arnica cream to reduce swelling, encourage efficient circulation and help the tissues to heal.

❧ Any damage to your Achilles tendon will take a considerable time to heal and therefore you should really wait at least three months before resuming an exercise programme. Even then, go cautiously, building up activity gradually and act promptly on any signals in the form of pain or discomfort.

TYPE OF SPORTS INJURY	GENERAL SYMPTOMS	WORSE FROM	BETTER FOR	REMEDY NAME
Initial phase of injury	- This remedy is a must at the first sign of pain, swelling and damage - It should be taken internally in tablet form and also applied locally in the form of a pain-relieving massage cream	- Jarring - Touch and pressure - Moving	- Rest	**Arnica**
Later stages of deep pain and bruising	- Pain is so great that it feels distracting - Injured area throbs and aches until a cool compress is applied	- Contact with heat - Touch	- Contact with anything cool - Moving	**Bellis perennis**
Later stages of injury where pain is worse for taking it easy	- This remedy follows Arnica very well if pain and discomfort is especially noticeable during or after a night's rest and generally much more comfortable for gentle, limbering up movement - Associated cramping pain in calf muscle	- Damp and cold conditions - Starting to move - Doing too much physical exercise - Keeping still for any length of time	- Warm bathing - Massage - Support to the damaged area - Not overdoing it	**Rhus tox**
Later stage of injury with deep, sore pains	- This remedy follows Arnica very well for the established stage of a tendon injury - Heel feels lame and heavy even though the initial swelling may have gone down in response to Arnica	- Going up or down stairs - Making too much physical effort	- Warmth - Massage	**Ruta**
Pains in damaged heel that are eased by raising the foot	- Severe aching and soreness left in the traumatised tendon - Episodic pain triggers alternate feelings of restlessness and exhaustion	- Resting the foot on the floor - Descending from a high step	- Elevating the foot	**Phytolacca**

homeopathy

●

41

tired, aching muscles

Anyone can get caught out by over-vigorous exercise that leaves you aching from head to foot the following day. Gardening after a winter's inactivity is often to blame, or taking up a racket sport, like squash and badminton that involve a lot of stretching and lunging movements.

practical self-help

❧ Learn to differentiate between the kind of aching that's coming from a muscle or group of muscles that have been temporarily over-challenged and a pain that's becoming a permanent feature of life. With the former, the muscles will become stronger and more flexible and therefore recover, while the latter is more likely to suggest a chronic problem in the making that would need some professional expertise. Consult an exercise coach, who can check that you are exercising correctly and/or a physiotherapist, who can suggest practical ways of counteracting the problem.

❧ Never be tempted to launch straight into a vigorous exercise session but always warm up the muscles first – a very large proportion of muscle strains occur as a result of cold, inflexible muscles being over-stretched.

❧ Exercise in an environment that is neither too hot nor too cold. Too hot and you will feel enervated and dehydrated very quickly; too cold and muscle cramps will very likely follow.

❧ Soak aching muscles in a warm bath of essential oils (chamomile, lavender, bergamot and rosemary oils are all very effective). Essential oils are extremely concentrated so add around four or five drops to the surface of the bath water after the hot tap has stopped running.

❧ After a warm bath, massage any remaining muscle aches and pains away with Arnica cream, continuing until it has been fully absorbed by the skin.

TYPE OF MUSCLE ACHING	GENERAL SYMPTOMS	WORSE FROM	BETTER FOR	REMEDY NAME
Typical aching that's been triggered by moving unfit muscles	- This remedy can be given routinely after any physical activity that's unusually strenuous - Muscles feel sore and bruised - Sensitivity can be so great that it's difficult to find a comfortable position in bed at night	- Moving - After rest - Jarring movement	- Lying down	**Arnica**
Aches and pains that feel eased for gentle movement	- Stiff, sore muscles that seize up after a night's rest - Aching can also cause restless, interrupted sleep because of the constant need to change position in an effort to get comfortable	- Staying still - Getting cold and damp - Too much movement	- Gentle motion - Warm bathing - Support to the aching area - Massage	**Rhus tox**
Aches and pains that are eased by pressure and rest	- Although light touch can feel unpleasant and painful, firm pressure to the aching part is temporarily soothing - Aching almost disappears when warm and comfortable in bed	- Slightest motion - Heat locally applied - Light touch	- Keeping still as much as possible - Rest	**Bryonia**

homeopathy

●

43

cramp

Cramp is what we call the intense, tight pain we feel when our muscles, often in the back of the calf and the back and front of the thigh go into spasm (involuntarily contract) either from a shortage of oxygen or a build up of lactic acid. Although not precisely a sports injury, a tendency to muscle cramp often accompanies exercise, particularly in hot or humid conditions where a lot of fluid has been lost through perspiring and not been replaced by drinking enough. Always make a point of taking a bottle of drinking water with you if you are exercising in high temperatures, working in extreme heat or taking a sauna.

practical self-help

> If you know you're especially vulnerable to muscle cramps, discourage any nutritional imbalances that can aggravate the problem by eating bananas, green leafy vegetables, wholegrains, fresh, unroasted nuts and seeds, and soya products. Specific nutrients, such as calcium, magnesium, potassium, and vitamins C, D and E also help. Opt for a good quality multivitamin and multimineral formula that gives you a good balance of the above.

> Periodical cramp that frequently causes trouble in bed at night is often related to high stress and tension levels. Therefore, stress-reducing forms of exercise, such as yoga, Pilates and Tai chi, which focus on relaxing each of the major muscle groups in turn, can do a great deal to solve the problem.

> Cramp often comes on when you have been standing or sitting in one position for a long time, of when you have been lying awkwardly in bed. In these situations, try to stretch the muscles involved gently, even though it feels difficult, holding it in the stretch position until the cramp stops and massaging all the time to increase blood supply to the muscles.

> We all experience muscle cramps at some point in our lives as they can happen at any time, when even the slightest movement that shortens a muscle triggers a contraction. However, cramps are most common when the body is ill-conditioned and susceptibility does increase with age due to normal muscle loss (atrophy) that begins between the age of forty and fifty. Preventative measures can certainly help and it is a good idea to practice regular flexibility exercises and always to warm up first with simple and controlled stretching.

TYPE OF CRAMP	GENERAL SYMPTOMS	WORSE FROM	BETTER FOR	REMEDY NAME
Cramping pains that follow an unusual amount of exercise	- Cramps can be accompanied by a general sense of muscle ache and pain that follows a punishing exercise session - This remedy is also specifically effective in banishing writers' cramp	- Motion - Touch	- Rest	**Arnica**
Muscle cramps that spring from an overall state of muscle tension	- This remedy is especially helpful when stress levels have rocketed off the scale - Tension and cramp settle in the large calf muscles and/or the soles of the feet	- Too much stress and tension - Relying on coffee, alcohol, cigarettes and stimulants to keep up the pace	- Rest and sound sleep - Peace and quiet in which to unwind and relax - As the day goes on	**Nux vomica**
Cramping pains that have a tendency to affect the left side of the body	- Muscles readily go into painful spasm and tremble and shake - Muscles generally feel knotted up and tense - Areas especially affected include the fingers, calf muscles and toes	- Too much physical effort and exertion - Going without sleep - Getting tense, angry and anxious - Hot weather	- Cold drinks - Putting a hand on the painful area - Massage	**Cuprum**

homeopathy

●

fainting

Sometimes referred to as 'passing out,' fainting can happen for a variety of reasons; for example as a result of severe fatigue or standing for an extended length of time, especially in hot weather. At the extreme end of the scale, fainting is a reaction to very bad shock or pain, although more often than not, it can be put down to low blood sugar levels, particularly during pregnancy. Symptoms are triggered by a short supply of blood to the brain that is usually caused by a sharp drop in blood pressure and are likely to include the following:

- **A buzzing sound in the ears with a general, progressive loss of hearing**
- **Blurred vision**
- **Feeling extremely dizzy and unable to keep a sense of balance**
- **Nausea**
- **Pale and drained complexion**
- **Feeling sweaty and clammy after coming round**

practical self-help

✂ Avoid drinking too much tea and coffee as these stimulants can trigger rapid, shallow breathing patterns that effect the levels of oxygen circulating in the bloodstream. Anyone concerned about their health should avoid having more than two cups of either a day.

✂ Always get up slowly from a crouching or sitting position or after lying down.

✂ If you have to stand in one place for a long time, flex your toes, contract and relax your calf muscles, and raise your heels up and down in order to stimulate circulation in the legs.

✂ If you have a tendency to low blood sugar levels and know you feel jittery, faint and lack concentration if you skip meals, eat a small, healthy snack every couple of hours. Where dizziness is an issue, also guard against low-grade dehydration.

✂ As soon as you recognise the symptoms of a faint, breathe steadily and deeply while sitting or lying down and, when you feel less light-headed, get up slowly and carefully.

✂ If you see someone has fainted, loosen any tight clothing around the neck and waist and encourage the patient to lie down with their feet very slightly raised as this will encourage blood to flow to the brain. However, if signs of distress develop, such as breathing difficulties or nausea, move them onto their side while you get medical help.

✂ If you feel shaky and distressed after a faint, place three or four drops of Rescue Remedy in the mouth, or dissolve in a small glass of water and sip at regular intervals.

TYPE OF FAINT	GENERAL SYMPTOMS	WORSE FROM	BETTER FOR	REMEDY NAME
Feeling dizzy or faint as a result of hearing bad news or seeing something upsetting	- Fearful before and following a faint, sometimes specifically focusing on death - Symptoms come on without warning and pass off quickly - Trembling and shaky with panic	- Becoming overheated - Fright - Becoming chilled	- Moderate, stable temperatures - Contact with fresh air	**Aconite**
Pale and clammy with a craving for cool air	- This remedy is most helpful when given after coming round - Classic fainting picture with pallor and sweaty skin that may feel chilly to the touch - Revives as a result of being fanned or having contact with cool, fresh air	- Becoming overheated - Overexertion - Lack of fresh air - Humidity	- After a short sleep - Fanning cool air over the face and head - Belching	**Carbo veg**
Fainting that comes on in a stuffy, crowded room	- Tends towards feeling chilly with specifically cold hands and feet, but also craves fresh, cool air - Vulnerable to fainting spells around the time of a period, in pregnancy or during menopause when flushes are combined with feeling dizzy	- Wearing too many clothes - Humid weather - Resting	- Loosening clothes or taking them off - Taking a gentle stroll in the fresh air	**Pulsatilla**

homeopathy

●

CAUTION!

IF ANY OF THE FOLLOWING SYMPTOMS DEVELOP AFTER COMING ROUND FROM A LOSS OF CONSCIOUSNESS, GET EMERGENCY MEDICAL HELP:

- **Reduction of movement in arms and/or legs**
- **Lack of strength in the limbs**
- **Tingling or numb sensations, especially if combined with any of the above**
- **Loss of, or slurred speech**
- **Noticeable disorientation and confusion**
- **Blurred vision**

nosebleeds

Nosebleeds are usually triggered by the delicate blood vessels inside the nose being ruptured, often as a result of blowing too hard with a tissue, or being hit in the face. Although they can look very dramatic, nosebleeds almost always look worse than they really are. An uncomplicated nosebleed shouldn't turn into a serious problem and almost all can be treated at home.

practical self-help

❧ Sit slightly forward or lean over a bowl or sink so that the blood will drain out of the nose rather than down the back of the throat. Breathe through the mouth as you pinch the soft part of the nose for ten minutes. If this only temporarily stops the bleeding, pinch once more for another five minutes. On no account lie down, and make a point of spitting out any blood that enters the mouth as otherwise it can cause nausea, vomiting and diarrhoea.

❧ Avoid blowing the nose vigorously for twenty-four hours after an uncomplicated nosebleed has occurred.

❧ Always keep your head above your heart as this will make your nose bleed less.

❧ Nosebleeds are often caused by dryness and are particularly common during the winter months when heated, indoor air dehydrates the nasal membranes. In order to prevent this, gently apply a little petroleum jelly to the inside of the nose and counteract the drying effects of central heating by using a humidifier at night in your bedroom.

CAUTION!

IF ANY OF THE FOLLOWING OCCUR, GET SWIFT MEDICAL ASSISTANCE:

- Bleeding that persists and refuses to respond to self-help measures
- Bleeding from the nose that is a consequence of a head or chest injury
- A nosebleed in anyone who suffers from a blood clotting disorder, or who is on medication that is designed make the blood less inclined to clot
- A tendency to recurrent, spontaneous nosebleeds should be investigated by your doctor

TYPE OF NOSEBLEED	GENERAL SYMPTOMS	WORSE FROM	BETTER FOR	REMEDY NAME
Nosebleeds that follow a minor fall or blow to the nose	- This is the general all-purpose remedy to give after any minor trauma has occurred as it helps minimise the psychological shock associated with an accident as well as promoting rapid re-absorption of blood from bruised tissues	- Being fussed over - Touch	- Taking it easy	**Arnica**
Profuse nosebleeds that are triggered during a cold by blowing the nose too vigorously	- During a cold the mucus that comes away from the nose when it's blown is thick, yellow and often blood-streaked - This can change to a gushing flow of blood after a hard blow of the nose - Anxiety often accompanies the sight of blood	- Inhaling cold air - Becoming chilled - Needing to make any sort of physical effort	- Calm reassurance - Being massaged	**Phosphorus**
Nosebleeds with a bright red, gushing flow	- Strong nausea that's worse for making even the slightest movement - Noticeable clammy, cold sweat with bleeding	- Moving even a little - Heat	- Keeping the head and body as still as possible - Contact with fresh air	**Ipecac**
Faint and dizzy with steadily oozing nosebleed	- Feels weak, wobbly and faint when nose bleeds - Face goes pale and skin feels chilly, clammy and sweaty to the touch - Yawns frequently from 'air hunger'	- Making any physical effort - Being in a stuffy room - Warmth in general	- Contact with fresh, cool air - Being fanned	**Carbo veg**

3 homeopathy and everyday problems

Common, mundane health niggles, while not serious in themselves, can still often be enough to make you feel low and run down. Within this context, effective short-term, homeopathic prescribing and sensible changes in lifestyle can do an enormous amount to give you back that *joie de vivre*. This chapter should also provide you with an excellent bridge between the more straightforward, routine prescribing to be found in the previous chapter on homeopathic first aid and the more individualised treatment relevant to this and later sections.

constipation

Going through a phase of stubborn constipation is really no joke, as the symptoms it sparks off can have a markedly dampening effect on your general sense of 'va-va-voom'. A one-off bout can be triggered by dehydration, especially in a hot climate where you may be losing a lot of fluid through perspiring, a diet that's become temporarily concentrated on refined, convenience foods and lacking in fresh vegetables and fruit, an escalation in stress levels, a lack of regular exercise or being on holiday, where the whole daily routine is changed, particularly in a new time zone. Constipation symptoms may include any of the following:

- **Bloating and discomfort in the abdomen**
- **Lots of wind, rumbling and gurgling in the stomach and/or gut**
- **A sense of incompletness on attempting a bowel movement, or absolutely no urge to pass a stool for several days**
- **Headaches**
- **Lack of appetite**
- **Tiredness and lack of 'sparkle'**

practical self-help

❧ Assess the quality of your diet and increase your intake of fibre-rich fresh fruit and vegetables straight away (bananas, plums, pears, apples and fresh figs, plus beans, pulses, wholegrains and wholemeal bread). A portion of stewed dried fruit with natural bio-yogurt is an excellent choice for breakfast.

❧ Drink six large glasses of filtered or still mineral water every day but avoid too many glasses of the fizzy variety as it both encourages abdominal bloating and aggravates a tendency to poor bone density and strength.

❧ Avoid regular use of laxatives. Although an occasional dose can be useful in getting things moving, there's a price to be paid for relying on medicines of this kind, even if they are made from herbal ingredients. Using laxatives on a daily or regular basis encourages the bowel to become progressively more 'lax' and once this tendency is well established, it becomes almost impossible to achieve a bowel movement without them.

❧ Don't put off the urge to go to the loo, however busy you happen to be at the time, for if you repeatedly ignore the signal that your bowel is ready to be emptied, you can find that the moment has passed and nothing much happens when you try.

❧ Avoid foods that can aggravate a general tendency to constipation, such as eggs, red meat and full-fat cheeses.

constipation in pregnancy

Constipation can plague women at any point during pregnancy and often causes particular discomfort and distress during the last trimester (the last three months before delivery). Anyone who has a general tendency to sluggish bowel movements will need to take extra care in pregnancy as not only can this nagging problem make you feel less than glowing with vitality but it can also lead to complications with haemmorhoids, which is something to avoid at all costs.

Any of the previous self-help measures should be useful for resolving an acute episode of constipation and all can safely be used side by side with any conventional support suggested by your doctor or obstetrician. However, established or very severe constipation in pregnancy that is linked to a long history of the condition will need treatment from an experienced practitioner.

CAUTION!

- If there is a noticeable change in your bowel habits that can't be put down to a corresponding in circumstances (like going on a different diet, or an increase in stress levels), it's worth checking the situation out with your doctor
- If bright red or dark and tarry bleeding occurs on passing a stool, get a prompt medical opinion

TYPE OF CONSTIPATION	GENERAL PROBEMS	WORSE FROM	BETTER FOR	REMEDY NAME
Constipation with lots of straining but little action	- This remedy is useful for full-blown constipation, or clearing the bowel when stool movements feel incomplete - Also useful if constipation follows a period of eating badly	- Touch - Motion - After sleeping	- Relaxing - Later in the day - Firm massage to the belly	**Nux vomica**
Stubborn constipation from neglecting to drink enough water. Completely lacking the urge to 'go'	- Bowel movements may be large, hard, dry and very difficult to pass - A severe headache can accompany constipation (also due to low-grade dehydration)	- Moving around - Lack of water - Warmth in any form	- Cool drinks - Resting and keeping as still as possible - Firm massage and pressure	**Bryonia**
Constipation that sets in as a result of a change in daily routine	- It's worth thinking of this remedy whenever constipation occurs when travelling - It can also help erratic bowel movements that follow an over-enthusiastic use of laxatives that results in alternating diarrhoea and constipation	- Stress - Cold food and drink - Emotional upset and anxiety - Tight clothing around the waist	- Gentle exercise - Loose, comfortable clothes - Warm food and drink	**Lycopodium**
Constipation with problems in passing a soft stool	- Constipation follows a general sense of sluggishness in the bowel – as a result, there's a lot of straining and even bleeding when attempting to pass a stool	- Too much starchy, low-fibre food - Lack of exercise	- Eating fibre-rich food - Warm food and drink	**Alumina**

homeopathy

53

cystitis

This is an unpleasant and painful problem that women are especially prone to. Infection is most likely to happen as a result of bacteria being transferred from the area around the anus to the opening of the urinary tract as the distance between the two openings is, proportionally speaking, quite small. Common symptoms can include any of the following:

- **A general sense of feeling under the weather and possibly feverishness**
- **Pain and burning at the beginning, middle and/or end of urinating**
- **Concentrated, strong-smelling, dark-coloured urine may contain streaks of blood**
- **A constant feeling of discomfort and/or heaviness in the bladder**

practical self-help

❧ Drink as much water as possible as this will make urine more dilute and easier to pass. Do not drink tea or coffee as these will only irritate the bladder further.

❧ Drink home-made barley water as this makes urine less acidic and therefore less painful to pass. Add two tablespoons of pearl barley to a litre of cold water and bring to the boil in a saucepan. Then strain off the liquid and cool before drinking. Don't be tempted to use commercially produced versions of barley water as these contain a hefty amount of sugar that can irritate rather than soothe the bladder.

❧ Cranberry juice or tablets can ease the pain and discomfort of an attack of cystitis by making urine more alkaline. Drink a small glass of cranberry juice as soon as the first twinge of discomfort sets in and repeat as for home-made barley water. If you are taking tablets, follow the recommended dose on the product label.

❧ Always wipe from front to back after passing a stool in order to avoid cross-infection.

❧ If you use a diaphragm and suffer from constant low-grade problems with cystitis it may be worth considering another form of contraception. Diaphragms have to fit very snuggly if they are going to be effective and can sometimes interfere with the free flow of urine from the bladder. Barrier contraception, such as a cap or diaphragm, can also encourage the growth of E. coli bacteria, which is a common cause of bladder infection.

CAUTION!

IF ANY OF THE FOLLOWING OCCUR, GET SWIFT MEDICAL ASSISTANCE:
- **If you notice deposits of blood in your urine**
- **If you develop symptoms of high fever, shivering, vomiting and/or severe pain in the sides of the body**

TYPE OF CYSTITIS	GENERAL SYMPTOMS	WORSE FROM	BETTER FOR	REMEDY NAME
Classic cystitis pain at the beginning, middle and end of urinating	- Burning sensations on urinating with a constant urge to pass water, however empty the bladder - Chilly, shivery sensations with fever	- Drinking coffee - Attempting to pass water when there's little in the bladder - Moving around	- Massage - Keeping warm - During the night	**Cantharis**
Cystitis with pain at the end of passing water	- Slight urinary incontinence with dribbling of urine while sitting - Symptoms may be more marked pre-menstrually	- Getting cold or damp - Exercise - During the night	- Standing	**Sarsparilla**
Cystitis that sets in after sex	- Stinging, burning pains on urination may be triggered by being catheterized for surgery, or after childbirth - Pains continue long after urine has been passed with a lingering sensation of being unable to empty the bladder completely	- Sex - Touch or pressure	- Rest - Warmth	**Staphysagria**
Cystitis with chilliness and restlessness	- All symptoms benefit temporarily from contact with warmth (such as a warm bath or cuddling a hot water bottle) - Severe burning sensations when passing water may trigger a feeling of anxiety	- Becoming chilled - During the night - Cold drinks - Alcohol - Making any physical effort	- Lying propped up in bed - Sips of warm drink - Company - Fresh air to the face and head	**Arsenicum album**

homeopathy

55

diarrhoea

This embarrassing and often debilitating problem can set in for a whole range of reasons, such as eating contaminated food and drink, or a diet that's too high in fibre, or because of stress and anxiety or over-enthusiastic use of laxatives. The symptoms are pretty unmistakable and may include any combination of the following with varying severity:

- **Cramping pains in the gut and abdomen**
- **Completely liquid or semi-formed stools**

practical self-help

❧ If diarrhoea has set in as a result of eating suspect food (strong candidates would be convenience foods that are past their sell-by date and salads and iced drinks in countries where the water supply is less than reliable), drink lots of fluid and don't feel obliged to eat if you don't feel hungry. Lack of appetite is generally a good sign, suggesting that the bowel is doing it's best to rid itself of undesirable bugs as fast as possible.

❧ Drink lots of water to replace the fluid that has been lost. This is especially important in hot climates in order to prevent dehydration from setting in and becomes an even greater priority if vomiting and diarrhoea occur together.

❧ When introducing foods again, avoid items that take time and effort to be broken down in the digestive tract. These include anything that has a high fat content, such as hard cheeses, red meat and anything that's been fried, or anything else that under normal circumstances you find indigestible.

❧ Eat foods that are known to be soothing to the stomach and gut, such as brown rice and homemade soups made with fresh vegetables and soothing spices such as ginger.

❧ If you know that your diarrhoea was caused by a stomach bug or eating contaminated food, avoid taking any medication that aims to slow down or stop the production of diarrhoea. This is important as blocking the evacuation of stools means that you hang on to the infection and feel worse for much longer than is necessary.

❧ The main emphasis should be on replacing body fluids, like water, but also essential salts like sodium and potassium, as well as an energy source such as glucose. There are also proprietary brands of electrolyte solution, which come as sachets of powder or effervescent tablets and simply need to be added to water. To begin with this should be taken as an occasional sip, slowly built up as the diarrhoea subsides.

❧ Do not take any tablets for headache or fever until the diarrhoea subsides.

TYPE OF DIARRHOEA	GENERAL PROBEMS	WORSE FROM	BETTER FOR	REMEDY NAME
Diarrhoea triggered by eating 'off' fruit or meat	- Incredibly weak, chilly and anxious with watery diarrhoea - Really fussy and restless even though feeling so drained - Sips of warm drinks ease stomach or abdominal cramps	- Becoming chilled - Cold drinks - At night - Being alone	- Contact with warmth in any form - Lying propped up in bed	**Arsenicum album**
Watery, profuse diarrhoea without cramping pains	- Lots of warning that a bout of diarrhoea is about to come on from loud gurgling sounds in the belly - Marked nausea, queasiness and weakness follow an episode of diarrhoea	- Just before, during and after an episode of diarrhoea - Eating - Motion	- Massage to the abdomen - Lying on the belly	**Podophyllum**
Painless diarrhoea as a result of feeling anxious	- Headachy, dizzy and generally physically exhausted and drained with loose stools - Becomes withdrawn and inward-looking when feeling ill	- Making any effort at all - Thinking of a coming stressful event	- Resting	**Gelsemium**
Diarrhoea with a craving for long drinks of cold water	- Unusually there may be no interruption in appetite between bouts of diarrhoea - Once an episode has passed (which involves lots of muscle cramps and straining) there's likely to be a marked clamminess and exhaustion	- Pressure around the waist - After drinking (although thirsty) - Moving about	- Rest - Being cosily wrapped up	**Veratrum album**

homeopathy

57

CAUTION!

IF ANY OF THE FOLLOWING OCCUR, GET SWIFT MEDICAL ASSISTANCE AS IT WOULD SUGGEST THAT DEHYDRATION HAS BECOME CRITICAL (TAKE PARTICULAR CARE IF THE PATIENT IS ELDERLY OR VERY YOUNG):

- **Drowsiness**
- **Severely reduced urine production**
- **Sunken eyes and/or very dry skin**
- **Noticeable drying up of body fluids such as saliva**

hangovers

After a very heavy night, many hangover sufferers say 'never again' with quite a lot of conviction only to find that, once the pain is a dim and distant memory, all their firm resolve vanishes into thin air! For all those repeat offenders, it can be a lifesaver to have some effective complementary strategies at hand to ease the situation and get the body back on track again as quickly as possible. The most common causes of a hangover are:

- **Drinking too much on an empty stomach or when overtired**
- **Having an unfortunate mixture of alcohol**
- **Women are likely to find that hormonal fluctuations affect the way in which their bodies react to alcohol. They have more fat deposits on their body than a man but little alcohol enters these cells because of their limited blood supply. Instead, their lean tissues (including the liver and brain) become affected by alcohol much more quickly than a man's and this effect is exaggerated at times of major hormonal shifts**
- **Low-grade dehydration can exaggerate the effects of alcohol**

If, despite your best efforts, you've still woken up with a raging hangover, there's still time to turn the situation around by doing the following:

practical self-help

❧ Drink a large glass of water at hourly intervals in order to re-hydrate the body as quickly as possible. This should help relieve some of the headache and nausea.

❧ If you feel you want something to eat, avoid fatty foods that only put extra strain on the liver. Opt instead for lighter items, such as a fresh fruit smoothie and wholemeal toast that won't overload the digestive tract.

❧ The herbal supplement milk thistle has a reputation for supporting the liver and helping the body detox more efficiently. The seeds have a protective action by assisting in cell renewal but should be avoided in pregnancy and in large doses. Follow the dosage advice on the product label.

❧ Rest and sleep are the best ways of allowing the body to recover, as they allow energy to be channeled into detox, rather than being diverted elsewhere.

❧ Adding a few drops of grapefruit essential oil to your bath should help the recovery process as this uplifting oil encourages the body to detox.

❧ If nausea and/or vomiting are a problem, sip a cup of warm fennel or ginger tea. However, if the headache is worse, wet a cotton wool bud with a drop or two of peppermint essential oil and run it gently around the hairline.

TYPE OF HANGOVER	GENERAL SYMPTOMS	WORSE FROM	BETTER FOR	REMEDY NAME
Classic hangovers from drinking too much alcohol when stressed	- Severe headache at the back of the head on waking which feels related to bad nausea - Vomiting is really distressing with lots of painful retching - Constipation makes general sense of feeling toxic more intense - Dizzy and on a mental and emotional short fuse with headache	- Cigarette smoke - First thing on waking - Lack of sleep - Coffee	- Sound sleep - Peace and quiet - As the day goes on	**Nux vomica**
Hangovers that have been made worse by low-grade dehydration	- Severe frontal headache with an extremely sensitive scalp - Even the slightest movement makes the pain and queasiness more intense, so there is an overwhelming instinct to keep as still as possible	- Bending forward - Becoming overheated - Eating - Lack of fluids	- Firm pressure to aching part of the body - Keeping as quiet and still as possible - Contact with cool open air	**Bryonia**
Hangovers that respond badly to drinking coffee	- Although commonly thought to be the cure for most hangover symptoms, this remedy is good for when a cup of coffee has the opposite effect - Accompanied by nervous exhaustion with a severe headache, characterised by sharp crushing pains	- Noise - Touch - Strong smells - Having to make a mental effort	- Warmth - Resting - Sound sleep	**Coffea**

homeopathy

59

bad breath

If this problem is infrequent, some of the practical self-help strategies listed below may be all that is needed to get things back on track once again. However, persistent problems with bad breath shouldn't be ignored as it can be the body's way of telling you about an underlying problem that demands attention. Possible triggers can include any of the following:

- **An upset stomach**
- **Dental problems such as cavities, or gum infections**
- **Dietary culprits can include any items that have a reputation for irritating the stomach such as spicy foods, drinking too much alcohol or strong coffee. Smoking cigarettes obviously doesn't help sweeten the breath either**
- **Recurrent sore throats, catarrh or sinus infections**

practical self-help

❧ Avoid dietary items that are known to aggravate this problem (such as those listed above) until the situation has cleared up.

❧ As a temporary solution, make up a natural mouthwash to sweeten the breath, especially if the throat is also sore. Add two drops of benzoin to a medium-sized cup of warm water and swill around the mouth. However, this is only the most stop gap of solutions as there's not much point in trying to cover up a deep-seated problem in this way for any length of time.

CAUTION!

If symptoms of bad breath are recurring frequently, get things checked out with your dentist and, if this doesn't solve the problem, consult your doctor

TYPE OF BAD BREATH	GENERAL SYMPTOMS	WORSE FROM	BETTER FOR	REMEDY NAME
Very bad breath that's linked to the presence of infected mucus	- This remedy can be especially helpful as a 'mopping up' operation following a throat or sinus infection - There's likely to be an excessive amount of saliva in the mouth with severe mouth and/or gum ulcers	- Becoming overheated (especially at night) - In the later stages of a cold	- Resting - Keeping a stable, ambient temperature	**Mercurius**
Bad breath that follows dental work	- This remedy is especially well-indicated where tissues in the mouth have been traumatised to the point of bleeding - Bad breath springs from the presence of blood in the mouth (e.g. after a tooth extraction)	- Touch - On waking from sleep	- Lying down	**Arnica**
Bad breath after eating too many rich, fatty foods	- The mouth is dry with a yellow-coated tongue - This can be the result of an upset digestive system or an established cold with infected mucus or catarrh	- Overly rich foods - Warm drinks - Before a period	- Contact with fresh, open air - Cool drinks	**Pulsatilla**
Bad breath from too much coffee, alcohol and/or smoking	- The whole system feels toxic as a result of high stress levels, too little sleep and a very unhealthy diet - The breath has a sour smell and is especially noticeable on waking	- Coffee - Alcohol - After eating - Being constipated	- As the day goes on	**Nux vomica**

homeopathy

loss of appetite

Losing your appetite on a short-term basis can happen for a whole host of reasons, which can include any of the following:

- **Catching a stomach bug that leads to low-grade uneasiness in the digestive tract**
- **Having too many late nights with not enough good-quality sleep**
- **Eating a disastrous combination of foods the night before that has taken a long time to be digested**
- **An excess of alcohol (or an unfortunate mixture of it), smoking too much and/or drinking too much strong coffee**
- **Fighting off an acute infection like a cold**
- **Emotional upset or anxiety**

practical self-help

❧ Before even considering a homeopathic remedy, look at the factors (listed above) that could be contributing to the problem and particularly avoid any of the food and drink that may have blunted the appetite in the first place.

❧ Fennel, ginger and peppermint teas will soothe the stomach and encourage efficient digestion.

❧ A short-term lack of appetite can sometimes be the body's way of telling us that energy needs to be diverted elsewhere in order to fight infection, for example, in the early stages of a cold. When this happens, drink frequent glasses of water to flush the system out as quickly as possible, and, if you get the odd twinge of hunger, avoid eating anything too heavy. Opt instead for foods that are easy on the digestive system, such as fruit juices, soups, fresh fruit and lightly cooked vegetables.

CAUTION!
IF ANY OF THE FOLLOWING OCCUR, CONSULT YOUR DOCTOR:
- **If there is no obvious reason for the loss of appetite and especially if it is combined with nausea, indigestion and/or weight loss**

TYPE OF LOSS OF APPETITE	GENERAL SYMPTOMS	WORSE FROM	BETTER FOR	REMEDY NAME
Loss of appetite from overindulgence	- Poor appetite with classic hangover symptoms, including nausea, headache and a need for peace and quiet - Irritable and grouchy with symptoms	- Eating - Lack of sleep - Too much coffee or spicy food	- Rest and sound sleep	**Nux vomica**
Loss of appetite from anxiety	- Poor appetite with rumbling, gurgling and some bloating	- Tight clothing - High fibre foods	- Loosening clothes around the waist - Passing wind	**Lycopodium**
Loss of appetite after emotional upset	- Temporary loss of appetite accompanied by a feeling of tension in the stomach	- Coffee - Alcohol - Smoking	- Eating small amounts often	**Ignatia**

homeopathy

indigestion

It can be misleading to talk about indigestion as one specific thing as it is a very broad term that can cover a wide variety of symptoms. These can differ greatly in intensity, and may include any of the following:

- **A sense of heaviness and/or bloating in the stomach**
- **Burping, or a feeling of wanting to burp**
- **Nausea**
- **Burning in the stomach or behind the breast bone**
- **If indigestion becomes really severe, acid may wash up into the throat**

Although an occasional bout of indigestion can turn up at any time and with no obvious reason, it is often brought on by eating on the run and especially by foods with a high fat content, or sprouts, onions, peppers and spicy dishes. Going too long between meals and then compensating by eating too much in one go is a common trigger, as well as eating a heavy meal late at night, which leads to indigestion in the early hours of the morning. Smoking and drinking strong tea, coffee and/or alcohol can also be responsible for irritating the stomach lining.

practical self-help

⊁ If you know that indigestion has followed a period of excessive eating and drinking, stick to foods that are friendly to the stomach for a while, such as brown rice cakes, non-acidic fruits (perfect examples are apples, pears, melons and plums), lightly cooked vegetables, salads, and small amounts of fish and/or poultry.

⊁ The liver plays a central role in good digestion and therefore it makes sense to take some of the pressure off it by having a few alcohol-free days.

⊁ Slippery elm food is good for the digestive tract as it forms a natural, soothing coating for the stomach and gut. If you don't fancy taking the powder mixed in a milky drink, there are also tablets, which include oils of peppermint, cinnamon and clove that help to release stubborn wind.

⊁ The process of smooth digestion begins when we chew food in the mouth and, therefore, it really is worth eating slowly in a relaxed setting.

TYPE OF INDIGESTION	GENERAL SYMPTOMS	WORSE FROM	BETTER FOR	REMEDY NAME
Eating too much fatty or rich food	- Discomfort and uneasiness in the stomach is more acute when walking quickly - There may be frequent 'repeating' with flavours of offending food temporarily recurring	- Too much red meat, cheese or cream - Lying down	- Walking gently in the fresh air	**Pulsatilla**
Eating too quickly or overindulgence	- Trapped wind that leads to burning and queasiness in the stomach - Acid may occasionally wash into the throat	- In the morning - After eating - Alcohol	- Burping - Contact with fresh air	**Carbo veg**
Feeling tense and anxious	- Acid indigestion is particularly noticeable at night, especially when lying flat in bed - Discomfort is temporarily soothed by sipping warm drinks	- High levels of stress and pressure - Cold drinks	- Being propped up in bed at night - Warmth in any form (drinks, or contact with a hot water bottle)	**Arsenicum album**

homeopathy

65

CAUTION!

An occasional bout of mild indigestion that sets in for obvious reasons is no cause for concern. However, if you are experiencing recurrent bouts after having previously been free of symptoms, it's worth seeing your doctor

minor infections

Nothing suggests quite so strongly that you are generally under par than going down with a string of minor infections. While these may not feel overly dramatic in themselves, such as a cold that refuses to clear up, they do indicate that your immune system is not functioning as efficiently as it should be. This situation can develop all too easily due to building stress levels, too little, or poor-quality sleep and a diet lacking in vital nutrients. In many cases, adopting the following self-help measures can be all that is required to break a negative cycle and help get your body's defences smartly back on track once again.

practical self-help

❧ Consider your recent diet, especially if you've been under a lot of stress and relying on quick-fix foods and coffee to keep up the pace. If this sounds familiar, switch to foods packed with antioxidant nutrients (Vitamins A, C, and E) that support the immune system by neutralising the effect of free radicals in the body and helping it resist infection, as well as preventing the signs of early ageing. As a basic guide, antioxidant foods are those that are bright red, orange, yellow or dark green in colour (broccoli, cauliflower, dark, green leafy vegetables, blueberries, apricots and kiwi fruit).

❧ Cut down on foods and drinks that have a free-radical promoting effect in the body, such as alcohol, and any fats that are classed as hydrogenated (these are vegetable fats that have been treated to remain solid at room temperature). Smoking should also be avoided as it depletes the body of essential vitamins (particularly Vitamin C) that help the body fight infection.

❧ If stress levels have been high, address them. According to research carried out at the University of Reading, positive, affirming experiences boost levels of circulating immune antibodies, while negative, unmanaged stress depletes them, leaving the body vulnerable to infection. It therefore makes sense to counter negative stress with a regular form of relaxation or aerobic exercise.

❧ The herbal supplement Echinacea provides really invaluable support in fighting minor infections as it can reduce the duration of an illness as well as prevent complications from developing, such as sinus or chest infections following a lingering cold.

❧ Make sure you get enough good quality sleep as during the hours of sound rest, all the major organs of the body work at a slower pace in order to to regenerate themselves. Depriving the body of regular sleep over a long-term basis also leaves the body vulnerable to recurrent, minor infections.

TYPE OF MINOR INFECTION	GENERAL SYMPTOMS	WORSE FROM	BETTER FOR	REMEDY NAME
Constant infections linked with very high stress levels	- This remedy is especially helpful in breaking a negative cycle of living in the fast lane with too little sleep and too much coffee, alcohol and junk food – it can give just the boost that's needed to get things back on track	- Lack of sleep - Noisy, unrelaxed conditions - Living on adrenalin rushes - First thing on waking	- Rest - Peace and quiet - Eating well and regularly - Later in the day	**Nux vomica**
Infections that are triggered by exposure to severe chill and dry, cold winds	- This remedy is most helpful in the initial stages of infection, especially if symptoms have come on very dramatically - Recurrent infections may be linked to a period of high anxiety	- Becoming chilled - During the night - Alcohol or coffee	- Sound rest - Fresh air	**Aconite**
Infections (especially recurrent urinary tract problems) that follow being emotionally hurt and angry	- When infections keep occurring after emotional trauma involving unexpressed anger, this remedy can stop the negative spiral - Minor suppressed niggles and resentment may briefly surface but this is by no means essential for the remedy to work well	- Dwelling on upsetting feelings - After sex - At night	- Resting - Contact with warmth	**Staphysagria**

CAUTION!

IF YOU FIND THAT YOU ARE UNCHARACTERISTICALLY PICKING UP ONE MINOR INFECTION AFTER ANOTHER AND IT'S COMBINED WITH THE FOLLOWING SYMPTOMS, CONSULT YOUR DOCTOR:

- Unexplained, persistent tiredness
- Significant weight loss for no obvious reason
- A general sense of being run down and in poor condition, combined with the appearance of boils or large spots

muscular aches and pains

If you're experiencing muscle twinges and you know this isn't the result of a recent injury or strain, your body is probably sending you a message that you're becoming physically unfit. It always helps to remember the phrase 'if you don't use it you lose it' with regard to achieving and maintaining physical fitness and strength. Our muscular system is like a piece of engineering that needs to be in regular use if it's going to remain in peak working order. If you underuse your body for a significant time, the muscle tissues will become weak and lacking in healthy tone; just think about what happens to anyone forced to stay in bed for a week to recover from a nasty bout of flu. In this situation the large muscle groups in the legs and arms lose bulk and strength within even a few days and it takes considerably longer to build that strength back up again. However, apart from a lack of regular exercise, additional reasons for generalised muscle aches and pains can include any of the following:

- **Straining poorly conditioned muscles by launching into an over-enthusiastic exercise programme without warming up first**
- **High levels of unaddressed stress and anxiety cause muscles, especially those in the jaw, neck, shoulder and back, to be held in a constant state of tension**
- **The early stage of a viral illness, such as flu**
- **A symptom of chronic illnesses, such as ME, chronic fatigue syndrome or fibromyalgia**
- **Residual muscle aches from a fall, long after the initial bruising has healed**

The following advice is aimed at easing generalised muscle aching that's due to being sedentary and unfit. Additional reasons (such as those listed above) are covered in other, relevant sections of this book.

practical self-help

❧ Your first priority should be to take up a form of exercise that will encourage your muscles to stretch, loosen up, and develop strength as well as stamina. Yoga is great for muscle strength, flexibility and stamina; Pilates encourages leaner muscle tone as well as building strength and flexibility and Tai chi is to be recommended if muscle aches are caused by high levels of tension and anxiety.

❧ However careful you are, exercise will make you ache quite a bit initially as immobile muscles are suddenly challenged to work. This sort of aching should feel low-grade and quite different to the sharp pain that follows a bad strain. The muscle twinges will ease of their own accord but you can speed up the process if you rub Arnica cream into the tender areas.

TYPE OF MUSCLE ACHE	GENERAL SYMPTOMS	WORSE FROM	BETTER FOR	REMEDY NAME
General aches and pains after overexertion	- Muscles feel bruised - Movement and effort of any kind is painful, - Finding a comfortable spot when resting in bed is difficult	- Moving - Touch - After sleep - Jarring	- Lying with the head lower than the body	**Arnica**
Muscles feel painfully tender when moved	- Aching muscles that feel much more comfortable for resting - This remedy is especially soothing to muscles that have been strained from overuse (e.g. chest muscles that become sore from repeated coughing)	- Deep breathing - Becoming overheated - Light touch	- Keeping as still as possible - Firm pressure to the painful area - Warmth applied to the painful part	**Bryonia**
Muscles that ache from cold, damp weather	- Initial movement is especially painful - Muscles become much more comfortable once they are limbered up - This remedy is good for rheumatic pains that come on as the weather turns cold	- Cold draughts of air - In bed at rest - Initial motion	- Warm baths or showers - Firm rubbing or massage to aching areas - Stretching	**Rhus tox**

homeopathy

tired all the time

This is one of the most common symptoms of modern life, if what I see on a daily basis in my homeopathic practice is anything to go by. The first step is to rule out any of the obvious health problems that can trigger a constant sense of lacklustre energy levels, such as an underactive thyroid gland, the after-effects of glandular fever, long-established sleep problems, anaemia, post-viral syndrome, depression and/or anxiety.

The practical complementary health advice given below will be helpful in lifting a bout of fatigue that is of relatively recent onset. However, if the persistent tiredness is associated with any of the conditions listed above, it would suggest that the illness is of a deep-seated chronic type and therefore it is a good idea to seek professional homeopathic support, in combination with conventional medical treatment.

practical self-help

❧ Assess the recent quality of your sleep. If it has become disturbed due to a temporary increase in stress levels, major changes in work or domestic routine, or dietary factors (such as an increase in coffee or alcohol intake) it's inevitable that you will pay a significant price in flagging energy levels. If this sounds likely, look at the advice given in the section on 'Changes in Sleep Pattern and Sleep Quality' on page 99.

❧ Make an honest assessment of your diet and the amount of stimulants that you regularly rely on. If you drink more than two cups of coffee, tea, and/or fizzy cola-type drinks a day, it's time to cut down, and if you also indulge in the odd chocolate biscuit or sugary doughnut with your daily espresso then it's particularly important to break the habit. Sugary foods will undeniably give you a temporary rush of energy but will also quickly leave you exhausted and craving more. Wildly fluctuating blood sugar levels make the pancreas work extra hard and create roller-coasting energy patterns. Opt instead for weak green tea that has a naturally low caffeine yield together with a snack that provides sustained energy release, such as unroasted nuts and dried fruit, and you can say goodbye to mood swings and lack of concentration.

❧ If feeling wrung out follows a nasty acute illnes or a period of unusually high stress, take a supplement of Co enzyme Q10. Sometimes referred to as 'the spark of life', this nutritional supplement can boost temporarily flagging energy levels in addition to supporting the immune system through its antiviral and antibacterial actions. The nutrient is present in mackerel, sardines, offal and peanuts and yet it is rarely therapeutically active in dietary sources alone. The best approach is to take a supplement of 30mg a day for a month if energy levels have taken a sudden nosedive.

TYPE OF TIREDNESS	GENERAL SYMPTOMS	WORSE FROM	BETTER FOR	REMEDY NAME
Profound exhaustion that follows an acute illness like flu	- A sense of never having felt back on form since the illness - Marked sense of droopiness and lack of sparkle (the eyelids may actually look droopy giving the face an exhausted look) - Headachey and dizzy or light-headed with lack of energy	- Becoming emotional - Making a physical effort - Smoking	- Rest - Sweating	**Gelsemium**
Tiredness that follows a period of high stress and hard living	- Lack of sleep is likely to be linked to an excessive intake of caffeine and too much adrenalin circulating in the system - Irritable, short-fused, headachey and grouchy with severe tiredness	- On waking - Alcohol - Eating badly	- As the day goes on - Having a regular, complete bowel movement - Peace and quiet - A chance to catch up on sleep	**Nux vomica**
Mental, emotional and physical exhaustion with a marked dip in libido	- This remedy is good for when demands build up and there's a general sense of not being able to cope - When shattered, moods fluctuate from total indifference to feeling as though about to snap	- Emotional pressure - After pregnancy - At, or leading up to, the menopause - Making love - Skipping meals	- Aerobic exercise (e.g. taking a brisk walk in the fresh air) - Resting	**Sepia**
Lack of energy from nervous exhaustion	- This remedy is good for building energy levels back up when there's an overwhelming sense of mental and physical weakness - This state may have been triggered by working too hard for exams or any other sort of intense, short-term pressure	- Anxiety - Too much excitement - Becoming chilled - Making love	- Sound sleep - Eating	**Kali phos**

homeopathy

●

thrush

The symptoms of thrush, or candidiasis as it is sometimes called, set in when the infective fungus candida albicans spreads outside the gut. Under normal circumstances, candida should stay within the confines of the gut quite happily but there are a number of reasons why this important balance can be disrupted. A course, or taking repeated courses, of antibiotics strips the gut of both good and bad bacteria, and the opportunistic candida can take this as an invitation to proliferate. Candida also thrives on a bad diet and being under intense stress can seriously diminish immune system functioning. The symptoms of a bout of thrush can vary in intensity and may include any combination on the following:

- **Vaginal itching**
- **Discomfort during sex**
- **A characteristic discharge which looks thick and white, not unlike cottage cheese**
- **Burning, itching and sensitivity of the vaginal area**

practical self-help

There are certain foods that encourage candida to proliferate. White sugar is the biggest culprit and so cut down on cakes, sweets and fizzy drinks. Savoury convenience foods (e.g. soups, baked beans, tomato sauces) also contain large amounts of sugar so try to eliminate these, as well as alcohol and any fermented foods, like vinegar (especially balsamic).

Take garlic supplements in a formula that has a high allicin yield (this is the active ingredient that gives garlic its therapeutic action). Continue for a week or so after the bout of thrush has cleared, starting again should it reoccur.

Natural, live yogurt, used as a topical application in the vagina, can feel soothing and cooling and also helps to restore a healthy pH balance.

If you have recently taken a course of antibiotics, the intestinal flora is likely to have been thrown into a state of disarray. Therefore, it is a good idea to restore the balance by taking a probiotic supplement; follow the instructions on the label.

Avoid wearing underwear made from synthetic materials as these can create a warm, moist environment in which candida thrives. Instead, choose natural fibres like cotton or silk that create a cooler effect.

Avoid using highly scented bath products that can aggravate itching and soreness during an episode of thrush. Try a salt bath or soak in an infusion of Calendula. Add one teaspoon of the dried herb to a cup of boiling water. Leave to stand for fifteen minutes, strain, cool and add it to your bathwater.

TYPE OF THRUSH	GENERAL SYMPTOMS	WORSE FROM	BETTER FOR	REMEDY NAME
Thrush that is particularly intense before a period	- Low back pain, chilliness and a noticeably urgent need to pass water - Burning sensation with vaginal discharge and lots of irritation and itching	- Moving around - During pregnancy - After sex - Touch - Becoming hot	- During the day - Fresh air	**Kali carb**
Low grade tendency to thrush that dates from pregnancy	- Thrush symptoms may be part and parcel of pre-menstrual syndrome, including headaches, severe weepiness and mood swings, and get much worse for becoming overheated - Vaginal discharge is thick and yellow-tinged	- Resting in bed - At night - Eating dairy foods	- Taking clothes off - Cool bathing - Contact with cool, fresh air - Gentle exercise in the fresh air	**Pulsatilla**
Painful, irritating thrush with noticeable vaginal dryness	- Thrush symptoms are accompanied by a characteristic vaginal discharge that is either thin and watery or jelly-like (rather like uncooked egg white) - Sex is especially difficult because of the vaginal dryness	- Before or after a period - Waking after sleep - Touch	- Holding a cool flannel against the sore area - Exposure to cool air - Being left in peace	**Natrum mur**
Thrush symptoms that appear at ovulation (mid-cycle)	- The vagina feels swollen, burning and painfully irritated - Discharges are characteristically thin and watery; even to the point where it can feel as though warm water is trickling down the thighs	- At mid-cycle or after a period - Touch	- Taking clothes off - In the evening	**Borax**

homeopathy

73

CAUTION!

- If symptoms don't clear up in response to the self-help measures within two or three days, it's appropriate to seek a medical opinion as your doctor may need to take a swab in order to confirm a diagnosis of thrush
- Don't be tempted to use a local, anesthetic cream in order to calm down the itching as this can mask an underlying infection that should be dealt with

wind

Although it's often regarded as a joke, especially when it has a tendency to travel noisily downwards, suffering an acute bout of wind doesn't feel very funny at all. The odd, one-off episode that's been triggered by specific unwise eating patterns can be dealt with speedily and effectively using a combination of the following complementary self-help measures. However, an unexplained or long-term tendency to wind production should be mentioned to your doctor. Common triggers of an acute episode of wind may include any of the following:

- **Eating beans, lentils, onion (especially raw), sprouts, cauliflower, peppers and cucumber**
- **Bolting food down very quickly, or eating on the run**
- **More ongoing, recurrent wind problems can be associated with chronic candida overgrowth. If this is the case, it is likely to be associated with distention and bloating of the abdomen**

Other possible conditions that can include a tendency to produce excess wind include irritable bowel syndrome and stubborn constipation (see page 51).

practical self-help

❧ If you're going through a noticeably windy phase, avoid any foods (listed above) that are likely to aggravate the situation.

❧ Choose foods that are easy to digest such as brown rice, lightly steamed vegetables and foods that are naturally low in saturated fat such as fish or the white meat of poultry.

❧ If you want to release trapped wind, sip a cup of ginger or fennel tea.

❧ If unwise eating habits have caused a recent bout of wind as well as a generally upset stomach, it may be helpful to take slippery elm food for a day or two until digestion settles down again. This can be taken as a milky drink or in tablet form.

The latter are especially good as they contain clove, cinnamon and peppermint oils that help release wind from the stomach or rectum.

❧ Avoid eating while being distracted as you are unlikely to chew food thoroughly when your mind is on something else. The process of smooth digestion starts in the mouth for the act of chewing breaks the food down into pieces that are small enough to be acted on by the stomach.

CAUTION!

If you experience ongoing problems with wind that are associated with unexplained nausea, lack of appetite and weight loss, this should be checked out by your doctor

TYPE OR CAUSE OF WIND	GENERAL SYMPTOMS	WORSE FROM	BETTER FOR	REMEDY NAME
Severe trapped wind with heavy, full feeling in the stomach	- Lots of swelling and bloating around the waist with wind that gets more noticeable after eating the smallest thing - Nausea and discomfort feel generally more intense for becoming overheated	- Tight clothes - Large amounts, or too rich food - Alcohol - Moving around	- Bringing up wind - Being fanned - Having a rest - Contact with cool, fresh air	**Carbo veg**
Wind as a result of overindulgence	- Severe wind and nausea accompany toxic feelings that are a hangover from excessive partying, drinking, smoking and overeating - Constipation may be at the root of digestive uneasiness with lots of straining but little result	- Too much stress - Lack of rest - Junk food - On getting up	- Sound sleep - Peace and quiet - Passing a complete bowel movement - Later in the day	**Nux vomica**
Wind from eating too much fatty food	- Queasiness and digestive discomfort are accompanied by ineffective burps with 'repeating' of flavours of foods eaten earlier - Wind pains are worse for jolting or jarring movements when walking on an uneven surface	- In the evening or overnight - Lying in bed - Warm food and drink	- Rubbing - Gentle exercise in the fresh air - Cold food and drink	**Pulsatilla**
Trapped wind with lots of abdominal bloating and noisy rumbling and gurgling	- Digestive discomfort is triggered by high anxiety levels or by eating too much dietary fibre (pulses, beans and wholemeal bread) - Severe flatulence travels noisily upwards and/or downwards	- Clothes with tight waistbands - Cold food and drink - Getting nervy about an up-coming event	- Being distracted from stress - Warm food and drink - Gentle exercise	**Lycopodium**
Wind with colicky pains in stomach	- Distention in belly with spasmodic wind pains that move from side to side - Burps smell like rotten eggs - Irritable and short-tempered with digestive discomfort	- During the night - Becoming chilled - Coffee - Alcohol - Touch - Lying in bed	- Regular, rhythmic motion - Warmth	**Chamomilla**

homeopathy

●

headaches and migraines

It's amazing how many factors can be responsible for triggering the misery of a headache, such as high levels of stress and tension, a lack of refreshing sleep, bad posture, emotional distress, dehydration, eyestrain etc. For the sake of brevity and convenience, the most common types of headaches can be divided into tension headaches that are related to tension in the muscles of the shoulders, neck, jaw, face and scalp, hangover headaches that follow a night of too much alcohol, particularly a mixture of beer, wine and spirits. (This is classed as a type of vascular headache due to the way that alcohol promotes widening of the blood vessels, causing a pounding type of pain) and migraines that involve a much more intense and distressing experience of feeling unwell. The range of symptoms that go with a classic migraine can include any of the following:

- **Visual disturbance with ziz-zag patterns and/or flashing lights around the margin of vision**
- **Nausea and/or vomiting, which may aggravate or ease the pain temporarily**
- **Severe pain that affects both sides of the head equally, is limited to one side, or moves from one side to the other**
- **A sense of the whole system being toxic for two or three days after the migraine**
- **Verbal disorientation and tingling on the face, lips or one side of the body**

practical self-help

✹ If you suspect poor posture is contributing to problems with recurrent headaches and especially if you are aware of tension in your neck and shoulders, consult an osteopath, chiropractor or Alexander Technique teacher.

✹ Eliminate coffee, tea, red and white wine, cheese and chocolate from your diet and see if the situation improves.

✹ Drink water as headaches are easily triggered by low-grade dehydration.

✹ During periods of high stress, it is essential that you get enough sound, refreshing sleep as this is a key trigger of tension headaches.

✹ Have a regular eye check up, especially if you are over forty when wearing reading glasses becomes almost inevitable, or if you are someone who reads a lot or spends a large proportion of the day at work in front of a VDU screen.

✹ Tension headaches and some migraines can be soothed by applying a drop of peppermint essential oil to a cotton wool bud and rubbing gently around the area of the hairline at the front of the scalp.

✹ If stress levels are high, substitute tea and coffee, which make you feel continuously wound-up due to their stimulant properties, with limeflower and chamomile herbal teas.

TYPE OF HEADACHE	GENERAL SYMPTOMS	WORSE FROM	BETTER FOR	REMEDY NAME
Throbbing headaches that come on as a result of low-grade dehydration	- Throbbing pains in the temples and very sensitive scalp are combined with constipation - Pains begin above the left eye and radiate to the nape of the neck - Mouth is dry and the system feels generally toxic	- Even the slightest movement - Bending forwards - Jarring movement, such as coughing - Eating - Physical effort	- Long, cold drinks - Resting in a cool room - Keeping the head and body as still as possible - Firm pressure to painful areas	**Bryonia**
Headaches that are triggered by low blood sugar levels	- Head feels tight and heavy with a woozy, dizzy feeling centred in the forehead - Disorientation is worse for stooping or bending forward	- In the middle of the morning - Making physical effort - Excessive amounts of sugary food and drink - Becoming overheated - Standing	- Contact with fresh air that doesn't chill - Gentle walking - Eating and drinking at regular intervals	**Sulphur**
Hangover headaches or migraines that come on after an excess of stress and pressure	- Sickening pains at the back of the head with a general sense of feeling disordered and toxic - Triggering factors include eating badly, an excess of alcohol, coffee and cigarettes combined with sleep deprivation	- In the morning - Waking from sleep - Stress and pressure - Being disturbed - Becoming chilled	- Peace and quiet - As the day goes on - Sleeping soundly - Warmth	**Nux vomica**

homeopathy

●

77

Homeopathic Support Table continued overleaf

TYPE OF HEADACHE	GENERAL SYMPTOMS	WORSE FROM	BETTER FOR	REMEDY NAME
Left-sided, pre-menstrual migraines	- Pains lodge above the left eye or move from the left to the right side of the head - Bursting, squeezing pains extend from the edge of the left eye to the side of the nose - Triggers include becoming too hot or overexposure to sunlight	- On waking from sleep - Leading up to a period - Alcohol - Becoming overheated - Feeling hemmed in	- Onset of a discharge (e.g. draining sinuses or flow of a period) - Contact with fresh air - Cool compresses applied to the painful area	**Lachesis**
Right-sided headaches brought on by being in hot, stuffy rooms	- Periodical headaches and migraines associated with hormonal shifts at puberty, pregnancy or menopause - Dizziness and nausea accompany headaches and are made more intense by lack of fresh air - Pulsating pains make the eyes water	- Resting - In the evenings - Around the time of a period - Eating a rich, fatty diet	- Taking a gentle stroll in the fresh air - Holding a cool compress against the painful part - Having a good cry on a sympathetic shoulder	**Pulsatilla**

CAUTION!

IF ANY OF THE FOLLOWING OCCUR, GET SWIFT MEDICAL ASSISTANCE:

- **A severe headache that is accompanied by vomiting, light sensitivity, stiffness in the neck and a high temperature**
- **Nausea, blurred vision and vomiting that occur together**
- **Nausea, head pain and drowsiness that set in after an accident or blow to the head**

IF ANY OF THE FOLLOWING OCCUR, CONSULT YOUR DOCTOR:

- **Headaches reoccur on a daily basis, especially if always present on waking**
- **Painkillers need to be taken on a frequent basis in order to keep headaches at bay**
- **Headaches last a whole day**

homeopathy and hormonal havoc

When our hormones are working optimally we should feel great as, with energy levels running smoothly and moods on an even keel we can enjoy a general sense of wellbeing. However, once they enter a state of imbalance a whole host of problems soon follow.

Many people associate hormonal problems with the menopause and increasing age and yet it is often negative lifestyle patterns that disrupt the body's natural rhythms and balancing mechanisms and compromise overall health for both men and women. The accumulative psychological effect of high, badly managed stress, poor nutrition and negative coping strategies, such as relying daily on caffeine, alcohol and junk foods, can seriously interfere with the endocrine system, which can trigger an overproduction of the adrenal hormones (especially cortisol and DHEA) and lead to symptoms such as cravings for sweets, weight gain, allergies, heart palpitations, insomnia, depression, fatigue, poor memory, foggy thinking, headaches, nervousness, inability to concentrate, recurrent infections and glucose intolerance.

Breaking the stress cycle is therefore essential and management strategies such as Tai Chi, yoga and relaxation, together with a healthy diet, are all good for counterbalancing the pressures that are now so much a part of modern life. This is the first step before prescribing any remedy as homeopathy will not be able to work to its full potential if negative lifestyle factors are allowed to maintain the status quo.

pre-menstrual syndrome

Problems with PMS tend to be experienced any time around or after ovulation (mid cycle), and often build as the onset of a period gets closer. Symptoms can be extremely wide-ranging and may include any combination of the following, in varying degrees of intensity:

- **Mood swings (including anxiety, tearfulness and irritability)**
- **Breast tenderness**
- **Fluid retention**
- **Food cravings (especially for sugar and/or salt)**
- **Disturbed sleep**
- **Problems in concentrating**
- **Abdominal bloating**

practical self-help

❧ Fluctuating blood sugar levels can aggravate the symptoms of PMS and therefore try not to go longer than two hours at a time without having something to eat. Choose forms of complex, unrefined carbohydrate that include essential fibre and encourage a slow, steady release of sugar. Foods that have a roller-coaster effect on blood sugar and should therefore be avoided include sweets, fizzy drinks, caffeine, cakes, biscuits, and alcohol.

❧ If fluid retention is a problem (sure signs include puffiness around the belly, fingers, ankles or feet), take care with your intake of salt. Apart from avoiding obvious sources, such as adding table salt at meal times, watch out for take-away dishes that contain large amounts of monosodium glutamate, salted crisps and nuts, and ready-made convenience foods.

❧ High stress levels have a negative impact on hormone imbalance as the adrenal glands are responsible for producing the sex hormones as well as the stress hormone adrenaline. If the body reaches a point where the adrenals are exhausted and overworked, symptoms of PMS are almost sure to be aggravated. In fact, the symptoms of exhausted adrenal glands are a very close parallel to those of PMS, including fatigue, mood swings, breast tenderness, and an inability to cope with stress.

❧ Take steps to reduce stress by making time to relax and unwind. Depending on the individual, this could take the form of daily meditation, progressive muscular relaxation, visualisation techniques, or soaking in a scented, candelit bath.

TYPE OF PMS	GENERAL SYMPTOMS	WORSE FROM	BETTER FOR	REMEDY NAME
Depressed and withdrawn before a period	- Salt cravings, headaches and/or migraines and fluid retention - Emotionally low and weepy - Noticeably clammy, cold sweats with bleeding	- Sympathy and attention - During and towards the end of a period	- Being outside in the fresh air - Gentle exercise	**Natrum mur**
PMS that builds steadily from mid-cycle to the onset of a period	- Severe mood swings, building steadily as the date of a period gets closer - Sleep disturbance, headaches and lots of cramping pain until the flow is established	- At mid-cycle - A late period	- Once the period gets under way - Gentle exercise	**Lachesis**
PMS with mental, physical and emotional exhaustion	- Moods shift significantly as a period is due, with a marked sense of being tense, stressed out, emotionally flat and unable to cope - Erratic blood sugar levels make all symptoms worse	- Emotional demands - Going for too long between meals	- Aerobic exercise - Having a small snack every couple of hours	**Sepia**

homeopathy

81

breast tenderness

Many women are familiar with a building sensation of breast tenderness as the date of their period gets closer. The degree of discomfort experienced can vary significantly from mild twinges to severe pain caused by jarring movements like running down a flight of stairs or turning over in bed.

Common symptoms that accompany breast tenderness and are influenced by the menstrual cycle include:

- **Breast enlargement; the difference can sometimes be as much as between a cup size or two and lasts until the period is well under way, or over**
- **A lumpy, fibrous feeling to the breast tissue that disappears once the period has finished**
- **Fluid retention; if this is the case, should be eased by passing noticeably larger quantities of urine than normal once the period is under way**
- **Breast tenderness and enlargement can also be related to taking prescription drugs, including synthetic female sex hormones such as the contraceptive pill or HRT**

practical self-help

❧ Certain dietary items have a reputation for aggravating problems with breast tenderness and, owing to the traces of artificial hormones that may be found in non-organic milk, it is a good idea to take care with dairy products. Caffeinated drinks can also aggravate problems as they obstruct the lymphatic system from draining efficiently.

❧ Always make sure that you are fitted for a bra rather than hoping for the best and squeezing into one that is the wrong size for you. The worst obstruction to eliminating breast tissue into the lymphatic system is a badly fitting underwired bra. If you are not sure of the correct bra size for you (especially with regard to the appropriate cup measurement), get professionally measured.

❧ If you use an antiperspirant, swap to using a naturally based deodorant instead. Although antiperspirants are convenient in keeping the underarm area dry, they do this at the price of sealing in sweat and this creates yet another obstacle to the lymphatic system, leading to discomfort and lumpy breast tissue. Although the UK studies done so far are too small to be conclusive, recent research has raised safety issues, due to the chemical parabens that antiperspirants contain (also to be found in cosmetics), as this may be linked to an increased risk of breast cancer. To find out about the latest research, go to the National Cancer Institute's site at www.cancer.gov.

TYPE OF BREAST PAIN	GENERAL SYMPTOMS	WORSE FROM	BETTER FOR	REMEDY NAME
Breast pain that is made more intense by the slightest motion	- Very tender breasts - Applying firm pressure during movement relieves pain; for example holding the breasts while running downstairs	- Low-grade dehydration - Turning over in bed	- Keeping as still as possible - Support from a well-fitting bra	**Bryonia**
Left-sided breast pain that gets progressively more intense from mid-cycle onwards	- Breast tenderness may only affect the left side, or be noticeably more acute on the left - The pain and congestion obviously diminish once the period gets well under way - Discomfort is aggravated for wearing restrictive clothing	- As the date of a period gets closer - On waking from sleep - Becoming overheated	- Loose clothes - Once a period begins	**Lachesis**
Severe pains with breasts that feel swollen and hard	- The right breast may be more affected than the left side - General sensation of restlessness and exhaustion accompany pain and discomfort, which may extend to the glands in the armpits	- Sitting up - Motion - At night - During a period	- Lying on belly - Lying on the left side - Resting	**Phytolacca**

CAUTION!

IF ANY OF THE FOLLOWING OCCUR, CONSULT YOUR DOCTOR:

- **Puckering of the skin on the breast**
- **Discharge from the nipple**
- **Awareness of a firm lump within the breast tissue or near the armpit**
- **Any perceptible change in the texture of breast tissue**

fluid retention

Fluid retention is not an exclusively female condition, although there is no doubt that women are more susceptible owing to their monthly cycles. Many find they are very prone to problems during the post-ovulatory phase and this is partly due to the shift away from oestrogen towards progesterone during this time, and partly due to pre-menstrual food cravings for salty items that can affect fluid balance in the body. Apart from hormonal fluctuations during a menstrual cycle, possible additional triggers may include a diet that's too high in salt, high blood pressure and low-grade dehydration. Common symptoms can include any of the following:

- **Puffiness around the eyes**
- **Swelling in the fingers, thighs, belly and feet and ankles**

Thankfully, if a tendency to fluid retention is menstrually related, the symptoms should resolve themselves once a period gets under way and the practical self-help section below will hopefully ease things through. However, more established problems will need professional attention from a trained complementary practitioner in order to rectify the underlying constitutional imbalance that may be triggering the chronic problem.

practical self-help

❧ Although the natural response to noticing symptoms of fluid retention might be to cut down on fluid intake, this is the worst possible course of action as the body would then react by conserving as much fluid as possible in the tissues, thereby making symptoms worse rather than better. Instead, drink five large glasses of water a day in order to flush out the kidneys and don't substitute any of these for a cup of tea or coffee.

❧ If drinking large quantities of water isn't enough to reduce minor symptoms of fluid retention, try adding fresh parsley as a garnish to your food as this has a gentle fluid-eliminating effect on the body.

❧ Pay attention to the amount of salt you are taking on a regular basis, as generous amounts of sodium in the diet are known to aggravate problems with fluid retention and high blood pressure. Be aware of 'hidden' salt to be found in some over-the-counter medications such as soluble painkillers and antacids and also in some mineral waters.

TYPE OF FLUID RETENTION	GENERAL SYMPTOMS	WORSE FROM	BETTER FOR	REMEDY NAME
Fluid retention with marked craving for salt	- Symptoms are noticeably more severe before or after a period - Marked thirst with very dry mouth and mucus membranes (e.g. in the nose and/or throat)	- Eating too much salty and/or fatty food - Becoming hot	- Contact with cool, fresh air - Sweating - Rest	**Natrum mur**
Rapid-developing fluid retention with marked puffiness of the skin	- Symptoms may come on as a result of a delayed period, perhaps as a result of trauma or stress - Skin on fingers and ankles feels tight - If this remedy works well, a large quantity of urine should be passed a short time after taking it	- Stuffy, overheated rooms - After sleep - Lying down	- Contact with cool air - Bathing affected parts with cool water - Getting up and moving about - Loosening clothes	**Apis**

homeopathy

85

CAUTION!

IF ANY OF THE FOLLOWING OCCUR, GET SWIFT MEDICAL ASSISTANCE:

- If severe fluid retention occurs in the last weeks of pregnancy
- If noticeable fluid retention symptoms occur in anyone suffering from kidney or heart disease

mood swings

Sex hormones are powerful chemicals and have a wide-ranging effect on the general sense of health and wellbeing that you are likely to experience on a day-to-day basis. While this is true to some degree for men (recent UK-based research tentatively concluded that males appear to go through a monthly cycle of hormonal change), so far it is generally accepted that women are more subject to significant physical, mental and emotional fluctuation.

Mood swings are part-and-parcel of these symptoms, and can occur mildly or with distressing and disturbing severity, depending on the individual. Because they tend to be associated with times of significant hormonal upheaval; puberty, during and following pregnancy, pre-menstrually and leading up to, and during, menopause, these are all times when women are susceptible. Common features of mood swings may include any of the following:

- **Rapid changes that move from euphoria to feeling emotionally low**
- **Tearfulness for no apparent reason**
- **Lack of mental focus and concentration**
- **Sudden onset of anxiety and/or jitteriness without any obvious cause**
- **Rapidly-descending feelings of irritability, anger or being on a very short emotional fuse**

practical self-help

❧ Feelings of jitteriness, lack of concentration and a generally volatile mood can be exaggerated by unstable blood sugar levels, which can also cause fuzzy-headedness, faintness, disorientation, palpitations and irritability. In order to stabilise blood sugar as much as possible, opt for foods that are known to give a sustained energy release such as brown rice, wholemeal bread, and pasta made from wholegrain flour, vegetable sticks and fresh fruit. Although the latter contains fruit sugar, this won't cause a sugar rush like refined, white table sugar that is released into the bloodstream much faster.

❧ Avoid drinks that can aggravate mood swings such as coffee and alcohol. The latter can be a problem because of its mood-enhancing qualities, which are fine when you feel good but a disaster if you're struggling to fend off feelings of anxiety or misery. Coffee also destabilises blood sugar and exaggerates irritability and jitteriness. Instead, go for soothing, mood-balancing blends of herbal tea that contain chamomile, citrus or valerian.

❧ Essential oils are great for restoring some much-needed equilibrium – you can vaporise a few drops in a custom-made oil burner, add ylang ylang (for lifting a low mood), grapefruit (for lack of focus and concentration), lemon (mental and emotional lack of oomph) and clary sage (helps balance a changeable mood) to your bathwater, or inhale their mood-balancing fragrance on a tissue or handkerchief.

TYPE OF MOOD SWING	GENERAL SYMPTOMS	WORSE FROM	BETTER FOR	REMEDY NAME
Volatile moods that build in intensity from mid-cycle onwards	- Moods shift rapidly from high to very low - Uncharacteristic fits of jealousy and insecurity, especially when pre-menstrual - As soon as tbe period starts, moods return to normal	- Ovulation onwards - After sleep - Delayed periods - Feeling hemmed in and overheated	- Once the period starts - Cool, airy conditions	**Lachesis**
Severe weepiness that acts as a helpful emotional release	- Bursts into tears at the drop of a hat, especially when shown sympathy and affection - Weepiness is the strongest feature of hugely changeable moods that emerge pre-menstrually, during or following pregnancy or the menopause	- Feeling neglected - During the evening and at night	- A good cry - Sympathy and attention - Having a gentle walk in the fresh air	**Pulsatilla**
'Hyper' mood alternates with feeling gloomy, especially before a period	- Mood swings are very intense if a period is late or missed altogether - Moves from irritability to anxiety and depression - Feels emotionally low, which aggravates exhaustion	- Alcohol - At night - Puberty and menopause - Skipping periods	- Being wrapped up warmly - Eating - Gentle exercise	**Cimicifuga**
Mood swings set off by a sense of being too stressed to cope	- General sense of mental, emotional and physical exhaustion leads to a non-existent libido - All commitments feel like unreasonable demands - This remedy is well indicated after too many pregnancies close together or during the menopause	- Skipping meals - Sex - Pre-menstrually - Being touched	- Exercise in the fresh air - Resting cosily in bed - After a sound sleep - Eating small amounts often	**Sepia**
Extreme irritability as a result of stress and not enough sleep	- Mood swings as a result of living in the fast lane for too long - Mental and emotional short fuse and difficulty switching off at night	- Too much coffee or alcohol - Smoking - Lack of sleep - Stress and pressure	- Sound sleep - Detoxing by getting the bowels moving	**Nux vomica**

homeopathy

irregular periods

There are predictable phases when you can expect a monthly cycle to go somewhat awry. Obvious times include puberty, when a regular menstrual cycle can take anything up to a year or more to establish itself, and leading up to the menopause. During the latter, it's very common for periods to either become longer, heavier and more frequent before they stop altogether, or to phase themselves out by becoming scantier. In between these two hormonal watersheds there are additional triggers that can lead to irregular periods:

- **Coming off the contraceptive pill**
- **Losing a significant amount of weight**
- **Excessive exercising combined with a very restrictive diet**
- **High stress levels for an extended period of time**
- **Following pregnancy**

practical self-help

❧ If periods have become irregular after being on an extreme weight-loss regime, consult a nutritional therapist to check that there are no deficiencies in your diet that are adversely effecting your hormonal balance. For example, large amounts of protein (from animal fat sources), sugar and saturated or transfatty acids can all interfere. Opt instead for foods that encourage a healthy balance, such as free range eggs, quinoa, small portions of lean meat, fish, beans and pulses, wholegrain cereals, tofu and broccoli.

❧ Periods that have become unpredictable after a significant emotional trauma, or from unusually high stress levels, can be addressed through stress management techniques.

❧ Rose essential oil has hormone balancing properties and can either be diluted in a carrier oil to make a soothing massage blend (four drops of essential oil to one tablespoon carrier oil) or added to a warm bath (no more than four or five drops).

❧ Especially frequent and heavy periods (to the point of flooding) are worth seeing a doctor about. If tiredness, palpitations and dizziness also accompany them, you should have a blood test in order to check for iron deficiency anaemia. Your doctor may also want to rule out the existence of fibroids, which are benign growths that can lead to heavy bleeding.

❧ If you feel that your periods have never quite settled down after coming off the contraceptive pill, consider seeing a trained homeopathic practitioner as they can prescribe constitutionally to re-establish long-term hormonal balance in your body.

TYPE OF IRREGULARITY	GENERAL SYMPTOMS	WORSE FROM	BETTER FOR	REMEDY NAME
Periods that are late to establish themselves around puberty	- This remedy is very good at encouraging the establishment of a regular monthly cycle where there may be a great deal of emotional ambivalence about the reality of periods starting	- After a period has finished - Displays of concern and attention - Being hugged	- Rest - Peace and privacy	**Natrum mur**
Periods that are slow to regulate themselves after pregnancy	- Periods may be intermittent and unpredictable after childbirth - Moods may also be changeable with a feeling of being constantly pre-menstrual, which takes the form of uncharacteristic weepiness	- Lack of sympathy and emotional support - When a period should be due	- Having a good cry - Gentle exercise in the fresh air	**Pulsatilla**
Irregular periods after a major shock or trauma	- Fast, unpredictable changes of mood from sadness and uncontrollable weepiness to laughter - When periods appear, they may be very scanty with an uncharacteristically dark-coloured flow	- Shock - Drinking coffee - Being touched	- Being alone - Relaxing breathing techniques - Having something small to eat at regular intervals	**Ignatia**

homeopathy

●

89

CAUTION!

IF ANY OF THE FOLLOWING OCCUR, CONSULT YOUR DOCTOR:

- **If irregular periods emerge for no obvious reason and do not return to normal for an extended period of time**
- **Any bleeding that occurs after the menopause has been completed**

heavy periods

As with irregular periods, there are specific phases in the reproductive cycle when women are going to be more susceptible to heavy menstrual bleeding. This is most common in puberty, when periods can initially be very heavy and/or painful, and leading up to the menopause, when the monthly flow can become unpredictable in timing and heavy to the point of flooding. Symptoms generally vary according to the severity and frequency with which heavy bleeding occurs but any combination of the following can occur:

- **Dizziness and light-headedness**
- **Fainting**
- **Nausea**
- **Flooding menstrual flow that often comes in uncontrollable gushes both day and night This can be severe enough to seep through double sanitary protection (such as using a tampon and back-up sanitary pad)**

Additional causes of unusually heavy bleeding include problems with fibroids, endometriosis or pelvic inflammatory disease. If all of these possibilities have been ruled out, but heavy bleeding still continues, medication may be prescribed in order to reduce the severity of the flow. For example, the contraceptive pill suppresses the natural menstrual cycle and stimulates a regular and lighter bleed.

practical self-help

➤ Heavy bleeding can be eased by adding a few drops of geranium, cypress or rose essential oils to a warm bath. For the maximum therapeutic effect, make sure you add four or five drops once the hot tap has stopped running and just before you get in.
➤ If borderline anaemia is causing complications through triggering symptoms of fatigue, palpitations and faintness, include plenty of iron-rich foods in your diet. Possibilities include eggs, green leafy vegetables, fish, wholegrain bread, seeds and molasses. It is important that your body absorbs the maximum amount of iron from these foods and so avoid drinking tea too close to a meal as it inhibits this action. Drink orange juice, which has a beneficial effect, instead.

TYPE OF HEAVY BLEEDING	GENERAL SYMPTOMS	WORSE FROM	BETTER FOR	REMEDY NAME
Heavy, gushing periods with severe nausea	- Profuse flow of blood alternates between steady oozing and gushing - Everything is aggravated by making even the slightest movement	- Overheated rooms - Any movement	- Contact with fresh, open air - Resting - Sips of cool drink	**Ipecac**
Heavy bleeding with severe dizziness and vertigo	- The flow is extremely dark and clotted as well as profuse - Because it is so heavy, anaemia-type symptoms are likely, such as weakness and fainting with buzzing in the ears	- Loss of fluid - Cold - Being outside in the fresh air	- Warmth - Bending double	**China**
Very heavy, dark, clotted flow	- Severe cramps precede the period by several days but once the heavy flow is well under way, the pain eases - This remedy is especially helpful in easing flooding, clotted periods at menopause with severe night sweats	- Waking from sleep - Becoming overheated - Alcohol - Standing	- Contact with fresh, open air - Cold drinks - Onset of the flow	**Lachesis**

homeopathy

●

abdominal bloating

A feeling of being bloated and distended around the belly and abdomen is a familiar sensation for most women at specific points in their menstrual cycle. The most common time is a few days before the onset of a period and is normally partly due to fluid retention (see page 84 for more details), and to digestive symptoms, such as constipation. All this contributes to a general sense of abdominal congestion where it is difficult to differentiate between the discomfort that's associated with the early muscular twinges of a period and that which is coming from a distended abdomen and is due to a sluggish bowel.

Abdominal bloating is also a symptom of irritable bowel syndrome and can affect both men and women. It is generally thought to be connected to high or unmanaged stress levels rather than the hormones, and its symptoms can include any of the following:

- **Uneasiness, rumbling and gurgling down the length of the digestive tract**
- **Frequent passage of wind in an upward and/or downward direction**
- **A general sense of inflation in the belly and abdomen that increases as the day progresses**
- **Bowel movements can alternate unpredictably between diarrhoea and constipation**

practical self-help

❧ If bloating becomes worse as a period gets closer, avoid salty snacks, convenience foods, tea, coffee and alcohol. The latter, in particular, have an undesirable diuretic effect; encouraging the body to conserve as much fluid in the tissues as possible.

❧ If bloating is associated with a sluggish bowel, have at least five portions of fresh fruit and vegetables every day, as well as five or six large glasses of still water.

❧ If abdominal bloating is associated with irregular, loose or only semi-formed bowel movements, cut down on foods that may be irritating the digestive tract. Items to approach with caution include too much bran, which passes through the gut too quickly, too many raw portions of fruit and vegetables (lightly steaming them is enough to make them more digestible), or excessive amounts of wholemeal cereals, pulses and beans. Eat foods that have a regularising effect on the digestive tract, such as brown rice, home-made soups, lightly cooked free-range eggs and a helping of natural bio-yogurt each day.

CAUTION!

- **If you experience a fever, puffy ankles that 'pit' when pressure is applied, or an inability to pass wind, stool and/or urine, together with fast-developing abdominal distention and pain, get prompt medical help**
- **If abdominal bloating occurs together with unexplained changes in bowel movements, and continues for more than a brief period of time, you should mention it to your doctor**

TYPE OF BLOATING	GENERAL SYMPTOMS	WORSE FROM	BETTER FOR	REMEDY NAME
Bloating of the belly with noisy rumbling and gurgling	- Severe bloating so that the waistband of clothing needs to be loosened by the afternoon or early evening - Distension is associated with a disturbed digestive tract that alternates between constipation and diarrhoea	- By the afternoon - Too much fibre in the diet - Anxiety, stress and tension - Tight clothing - Eating	- Loosening clothes - Sips of warm drink - Burping - Passing water	**Lycopodium**
Pre-menstrual bloating that builds from ovulation onwards	- Sense of bloating and tension in the belly and abdomen eases as soon as the flow starts - A tendency to pre-menstrual constipation can add to the general sense of abdominal discomfort and congestion	- Any tight clothing that presses on the waist - After sleep - Delayed period - Alcohol	- Contact with fresh, cool air - Onset of a period - Cold drinks - Eating	**Lachesis**
Bloating with stubborn constipation and/or fluid retention	- Colicky pains with distension are eased by passing wind - Constipation may occur on alternate days with a sense of inactivity in the rectum	- Cravings for salty snacks or fatty foods - Eating - After a period - Pressure - Being fussed over	- Contact with fresh, cool air - Tight clothes - Skipping meals - Massaging the affected area	**Natrum mur**
Bloating from severe trapped wind in stomach and gut	- Eating even the smallest portion of food makes the discomfort of bloating more severe - Symptoms are much more noticeable when lying down and a little easier when bending over	- Overindulgence - Becoming overheated - Pressure of clothes	- Passing wind - Fanning the face and head with cool air	**Carbo veg**

homeopathy

93

food cravings

Women generally experience more food cravings than men as they are an extremely common feature of pre-menstrual syndrome. Indeed, sometimes the cravings for chocolate or crisps are so strong that a packet of biscuits or an extra large packet of nuts can easily disappear all in one go! Additional times when food cravings can attack include:

- **Periods of high stress and tension when the simple act of eating and drinking provides a sense of comfort**
- **When a dependence on caffeine or sweet things has been established in an effort to get through the day**
- **Yo-yo dieting an often creates a craving for certain foods, simply because they are forbidden and theoretically out of reach**

practical self-help

❧ Seemingly innocuous substances, like sugar, salt and caffeinated drinks are addictive and therefore it is a bad idea to incorporate them into your daily routine. The standard pattern for dependency is to start craving for increasingly larger and more frequent quantities in order to gain the 'lift' that is part and parcel of the experience.

❧ Like kicking any bad habit, it's best to resolve to stop completely as half measures are almost always doomed to failure. For the most successful results, make sure you have alternative healthy snacks on hand so that you don't feel completely deprived and tempted to take a retrograde step. Eat a small snack every couple of hours so you don't experience gnawing hunger and the urge to grab a bag of crisps as a quick fix to fill the gap.

❧ Food cravings, like the need for a cigarette, are often linked to nervous energy and the physical need to do something with your hands. If this is the case, have healthy snacks close by, such as fresh sunflower seeds, unsalted nuts such as Brazils, almonds, and walnuts (all beneficial sources of essential fatty acids that can encourage optimum hormone balance) and small helpings of dried fruit.

❧ If stress levels are very high, go for a brief walk in the fresh air rather than taking refuge in a cup of coffee and a Danish pastry. If you also drink a cup of green tea with a healthy snack, you'll feel clear-headed and energised rather than sluggish and guilty.

CAUTION!

If you experience a craving for sweet foods in combination with an unquenchable thirst, increased urine output and fatigue, you should consult your doctor and have your blood sugar levels tested

TYPE OF CRAVING	GENERAL SYMPTOMS	WORSE FROM	BETTER FOR	REMEDY NAME
Cravings for coffee and alcohol to keep the pace up when under stress	- As stress levels rise, so do the food cravings, leading to snappishness, an inablility to relax, problems with concentration and disturbed sleep - If this goes on long enough, poor appetite, indigestion, constipation and tension headaches are likely to develop	- Lack of sleep - Too many stimulants - Relying on painkillers - Excitement	- Getting sound sleep - Peace and quiet - Later in the day	**Nux vomica**
Marked pre-menstrual cravings for salt	- The low, withdrawn mood that descends before a period encourages comfort eating, aggravating fluid retention and a sense of guilt	- During and after a period - Emotional release - Eating - Becoming overheated	- Being left alone - Skipping meals - Gentle exercise	**Natrum mur**
Cravings for ice cream and sweet carbohydrates	- Cravings for carbohydrates can emerge with a vengeance in the run up to the menopause - Tired and exhausted with a tendency to feel the whole system is sluggish. As a result, weight gain can become a real problem	- Making any physical effort - Feeling anxious - Mental strain and pressure	- When constipated - Resting - Massage	**Calc carb**
Cravings for sugary things when tense and anxious	- Although the craving for sugar in any form (fizzy drinks, sweets, chocolate etc.) is very strong, the reaction to eating it is to make the situation worse - Digestive upsets (nausea and nervous diarrhoea) are aggravated by sugary foods	- Anticipating a stressful event - Crowds - Cold, sweet foods (e.g. ice cream or puddings) - Before a period	- Contact with cool, fresh air - Moving about - Burping	**Arg nit**

homeopathy

hot flushes

It's been estimated that approximately 70 per cent of menopausal women experience some degree of difficulty with hot flushes. However, it's also important to stress that hot flushes are by no means inevitable and if they do begin to cause problems, there is a wealth of practical tips to improve the situation quickly and effectively. Common symptoms of hot flushes can include any of the following:

- **A sudden and general sense of heat that moves up from the feet or the waist**
- **A feeling of uneasiness or foreboding before a flush appears**
- **As the heat builds it is likely to be broken by a sweat. This may continue to feel hot, or may move on to a cold, chilled, clammy feeling**
- **After the flush there may be a powerful sense of exhaustion**

practical self-help

✂ Since hot flushes are usually triggered by the ovaries producing less and less oestrogen at menopause, take advantage of the natural plant-based oestrogens present in all soya. Importantly, these phyto-oestrogens appear to have none of the drawbacks of the synthetic oestrogen in conventional hormone replacement therapy.

✂ Synthetic clothing fibres encourage the body to hold its heat, so wear clothes made from cotton, linen or silk, which allow the skin to breathe.

✂ Layer your clothes so that you can easily cool yourself down at the first sign of a flush, and warm up again once the chilled feeling sets in.

✂ Avoid alcohol, coffee and other caffeinated drinks and spicy foods that have a reputation for triggering or aggravating hot flushes.

✂ Regular exercise discourages problems with hot flushes by reducing the tendency to anxiety and tension and maintaining efficient circulation. Choose from cycling, power walking, yoga, swimming or cycling.

✂ Significant reserves of oestrogen are stored in fatty tissue and therefore being underweight can aggravate problems with hot flushes – gaining anything up to an extra 7lb at menopause can even be positively helpful. However, carrying excessive weight isn't healthy either so don't overdo it!

TYPE OF HOT FLUSH	GENERAL SYMPTOMS	WORSE FROM	BETTER FOR	REMEDY NAME
Hot flushes that come on in overheated rooms	- Although flushes are frequent, there may be a general sense of feeling chilly at other times	- Weepy and emotional with flushes - Lack of fresh air - Hot drinks	- Walking outside - Cold drinks	**Pulsatilla**
Hot flushes that are preceded by a sense of anxiety	- Flushes and sweats are incredibly hot and can feel as though the body is being splashed with hot water - Feeling under stress, anxious or emotional can trigger a flush	- Anger or excitement - Becoming chilled	- Relaxation - Reassurance	**Phosphorus**
Hot flushes that come on after sleep	- Flushes can be triggered by feeling hemmed in or wearing clothes that feel restrictive (e.g. a polo neck sweater or a scarf)	- Contact with heat - Warm baths - Being in the sun	- Loose clothes - Cold drinks - Onset of a period	**Lachesis**

homeopathy for mid-life and beyond

These days, Botox, cosmetic surgery and chemical peels are no longer the concern of just the rich and famous as growing numbers decide, as they get older, to have 'enhancement' procedures of some kind. While focusing on improving the externals in this way is quite understandable, this is by no means the only answer to looking youthful. In fact, there is little point in having a few lines and crinkles temporarily ironed out if you feel exhausted and your libido seems to have gone AWOL.

More and more evidence suggests that good emotional and physical health is far more important than all the surgery that money can buy as the emphasis falls on looking as young or old as you *feel*. And this is precisely why complementary medicine is so invaluable, for it can help solve many of the common problems that surface at mid-life safely and holistically. This chapter will give you the basic tools you need in order to keep your body strong, supple and in good health so you can take whatever the future has in store for you, and run with it.

changes in sleep pattern and sleep quality

A sound, refreshing night's sleep is one the best anti-ageing weapons you have at your disposal and yet, sadly, it's also one of the things that has a tendency to go west as we get older. There can be a variety of reasons for this which may include any of the following:

- Hormonal changes that occur premenstrually and in the run up to the menopause
- Physical symptoms of the menopause, such as night sweats, can make it harder to drift off and stay asleep
- Health problems, such as an over-active thyroid gland, anxiety, depression, ME, eczema and asthma
- The body's digestive functions becoming slower and less efficient with age. In some cases, this can be due to a chronic problem, such as a hiatus hernia or a tendency to recurrent heartburn and indigestion
- High, unmanaged stress levels can make it hard both to switch off at the end of a day and establish an irritating pattern of frequent or early waking

If your sleep is regularly disturbed, it is very important to take action as the problems associated with sleep deprivation are well documented and can include any of the following:

- **Mood swings**
- **Mental and physical fatigue**
- **Signs of premature ageing**
- **Irritability**
- **Recurrent, minor infections**
- **Poor concentration**

It is natural that changes in your sleep pattern will emerge over the years. By the age of 70, an average night's rest generally consists of fewer than seven hours and is a far cry from a newborn baby, who can sleep 18 hours out of every 24. The self-help advice that follows is excellent for getting a wayward sleep pattern back on track and should also help improve the depth and quality of sleep for anyone who feels short-changed in the rest department on a more ongoing basis.

practical self-help

❧ Check your diet for stimulating, caffeine-based substances and don't forget that there can be some surprises in green tea, hot chocolate, painkillers and some over-the-counter cold medicines. Have no more than two cups of caffeinated drinks a day, and always avoid having any after 4p.m. in the afternoon.

❧ Eating a heavy meal late at night makes it harder to get comfortable and drift off to sleep. The digestive organs work slower when the body is resting and so breaking down a rich meal obviously takes longer and involves more effort; often leading to indigestion, nausea or heartburn. Avoid eating a large meal after 8p.m. and, if you don't have a choice, go for easily digested foods such as fish, vegetables and poultry.

❧ Some foods and drinks have sedative, relaxing properties and therefore are a good choice for a late night snack. A warm milky drink makes an ideal nightcap, as well as foods that have a high tryptophan content, such as bananas, avocado or peanut butter.

❧ Don't be tempted to have a stiff drink in order to relax. Alcohol might knock you out quickly but it will not help you to a refreshing level of sleep and there is a strong chance you will wake early, feeling sluggish.

❧ Instead of alcohol, choose a sleep-inducing herbal tea, such as chamomile, or a blend that contains valerian, passiflora and lemon balm.

❧ If you need a temporary prop to help you through a bad period and want to avoid conventional sleeping tablets, try the Avena sativa compound. This is made from a herbal tincture of hops and passiflora to which a homeopathic dilution of Coffea has been added, and you simply take a few drops diluted in a small glass of water before bed.

TYPE OF SLEEP PROBLEM	GENERAL SYMPTOMS	WORSE FROM	BETTER FOR	REMEDY NAME
Jittery and sleepless at night from drinking too much coffee	- The body feels tired but there's likely to be a rush of ideas going through the mind - Very sensitive to the slightest sound which can disturb a light, fitful sleep - Very irritable when wakeful	- The slightest noise - Becoming chilled - Alcohol - Excitement	- Becoming comfortably warm - Getting sound sleep	**Coffea**
Sleep that is disturbed by severe night sweats	- Very irritable when wakeful - Hot and anxious in bed - Palpitations accompany night sweats, with a tendency to jerk awake just when dropping off to sleep - Aversion to going to bed	- Delayed menstruation - On first waking - Becoming overheated - Alcohol	- Contact with cool air - Onset of a period - Sipping cool drinks	**Lachesis**
Disturbed sleep as a result of overindulgence	- System feels toxic - Wakes in the early hours feeling wide awake, then falls into a deep sleep when it's time to get up	- Too much food, alcohol and/or coffee - Sedentary habits - Overexcitement	- Having a nap - Rest - Peace and quiet	**Nux vomica**
Disturbed sleep from needing to pass water frequently at night	- Tosses and turns all night - Pulls covers up and down all night - Wakes confused and drowsy	- Becoming overheated - Lying on back (pressure on bladder) - Eating fatty, rich foods late at night	- Contact with cool, fresh air - Taking gentle exercise out of doors - Taking clothes off	**Pulsatilla**

homeopathy

●

101

Homeopathic Support continued overleaf

TYPE OF SLEEP PROBLEM CONT..	GENERAL SYMPTOMS	WORSE FROM	BETTER FOR	REMEDY NAME
Disturbed sleep pattern that dates from bereavement	- Tosses, turns and yawns and gets very frustrated when unable to sleep - Nasty sense of jerky limbs - Sleeps so lightly hears every sound	- Too much coffee - Being touched - Smoking - Becoming chilled	- Moving around - Passing water - Breathing deeply - Eating a light snack	**Ignatia**
Difficulty sleeping as a result of restless legs	- Problems with sleep can set in after being under considerable emotional strain (e.g. nursing a sick partner) - Distress takes the form of constantly moving arms and legs during light sleep with possible cramping pains	- Exposure to dry cold winds - Extreme changes of temperature - Caffeinated drinks	- Sipping a cold drink - Feeling warm in bed	**Causticum**

CAUTION!

IF ANY OF THE FOLLOWING OCCUR, CONSULT YOUR DOCTOR:

• If sleep problems are associated with a more chronic condition, such as severe anxiety and/or depression

• Sleeplessness that is associated with severe menopausal symptoms in women or prostate problems in men

night sweats

Night sweats are a continuation of hot flushes and while they may not be the sole cause of the sleep problems that emerge for many women at mid-life, they are certainly a co-factor that make sleep feel more elusive and less satisfying. In common with hot flushes, night sweats generally occur in the phase called peri-menopause, which is the time when menopausal symptoms, such as irregular periods, changes in body temperature and fluctuations in energy, are a feature of daily life until menopause has been achieved and periods stop altogether. This process can take anything up to eight or more years but you can expect most women to have reached the menopause by their early fifties.

Night sweats and hot flushes are triggered by the body's thermostat being temporarily unable to keep a state of balanced temperature. As a result, women who suffer frequent or severe night sweats can feel as though they are hauling the covers up and down all night in an effort to cool down, or warm up.

Common symptoms of nights sweats can include any of the following:

- **Sweats that especially affect the head, between the breasts, under the arms, the back, and around the waist or those that are experienced as more of a sweaty sensation across the whole body**
- **The nature and severity of the sweats can vary hugely; some drench so thoroughly that you have to get up and change sheets and nightclothes, while others cause only mild discomfort and afterwards you can simply turn over and go back to sleep**
- **Palpitations and a feeling of foreboding or anxiety often precede a night sweat**
- **Many night sweats reach their peak in the hours just before rising; women report that they wake just before a sweat breaks and at the time when they are due to get up**

Conventional medical treatment focuses on the use of Hormone Replacement Therapy, which supplies the body with synthetic oestrogen and/or progestogen, the theory being that hot flushes and night sweats are symptoms of the declining female sex hormones in a woman's body at mid-life. While this is undoubtedly the case, questions have been raised over the last five years about the safety issues concerning this form of treatment. In the US, high-profile studies involving combination hormone therapy, oestrogen plus progestagen, had to be halted because of results that indicated it increased the risk of breast cancer, heart disease, stroke and blood clots.

Controversy continues but generally most conventional doctors advise against any long-term use of HRT (ideally no more than five years if possible, or a maximum of ten) and recommend complementary medical treatment for mild to moderate symptoms. In addition, making healthy lifestyle changes can improve your circulatory health and therefore it is a good idea to take regular moderate exercise, cut down drastically on red meat and other saturated fats and give up smoking once and for all.

Bear in mind that when you are considering conventional or complementary treatments it really doesn't have to be a strict either/or dilemma. Homeopathic remedies can be used exclusively, side-by-side with HRT or as a support that allows you to come off HRT without the pressure of going completely 'cold turkey'.

practical self-help

❧ Sage and Black cohosh are the herbal alternatives to HRT, and appear to be without the potential side effects. They are obtainable in tincture or tablet form and, while both appear to ease menopausal hot flushes and night sweats, black cohosh also usefully reduces vaginal dryness that is often a key feature of menopausal symptoms.

❧ Specific foods can aggravate a tendency to produce night sweats and therefore alcohol, tea, coffee and spicy foods are all best avoided or taken in strict moderation.

❧ Eating patterns also have an impact on night sweats and therefore it can help to have a light, healthy snack before bed to ensure that blood sugar levels don't plummet overnight. For advice on good foods that will encourage a sound night's rest, see the section on 'Changes In Sleep Pattern And Sleep Quality' on page 99.

❧ Keep your bedroom comfortably cool and well ventilated (although not too much like a fridge as severe chills can set in after a hot sweat). In summer, when it is especially hot, you may find it helpful to use a fan but make sure it rotates as otherwise it can create a chilled effect on the skin.

❧ Nightclothes, if you choose to wear them, should be made from natural fibres, such as cotton or silk, as these allow the skin to breathe and stay as cool as possible. Avoid synthetic fibres like nylon polyester and microfibres that trap the heat in and make you more susceptible to night sweats.

❧ Keep a bowl of cool water, a sponge, towel and dry change of nightclothes by the side of your bed if you know you're prone to drenching sweats. This avoids the upheaval of having to get up in the middle of the night and find what you need in the dark and will almost certainly make it easier for you to get back to sleep.

TYPE OF NIGHT SWEAT	GENERAL SYMPTOMS	WORSE FROM	BETTER FOR	REMEDY NAME
Violent night sweats that prevent sleep and cause severe fatigue during the day	- Wakes drenched in sweat with pulsations of heat coursing through the body - Feels mentally, emotionally and physically drained all the time as a result of sleep deprivation	- After sex - After first falling asleep - Massage - Feeling under pressure of living up to the expectations of others	- Vigorous aerobic workouts - Becoming warm in bed - After a sound, refreshing sleep - Cool bathing	**Sepia**
Severe night sweats with anxiety and rapid heartbeat that come on when waking	- Extreme sensitivity to becoming overheated at night; bedrooms need to be kept cool and well aired - Marked aversion to any restriction around the neck or waist from bedcovers or nightwear	- On first waking - Slight touch or pressure - Hot drinks - Alcohol	- Contact with fresh air - Cool bathing and cool compresses - Sipping cold drinks	**Lachesis**
Night sweats that make it almost impossible to get comfortable at night	- Wakes confused and disoriented as a result of light, fitful sleep - Feels chilly at intervals through the night but dislikes warm and stuffy rooms - Becomes emotional as a result of constantly interrupted sleep	- Contact with warm air - Resting in bed - Eating rich food late at night - In the evening before going to bed	- Gentle exercise in the fresh air that doesn't result in becoming overheated - Massage - Lying with the head elevated	**Pulsatilla**
Extreme heat with sweats that can only be cooled down by pushing the feet outside the bedcovers	- Distressing sensitivity to heat that triggers sudden flushes followed by severe chills - Skin feels as though it is burning but stays dry - Exhausted and drained after a sweat	- Making too much physical effort - Becoming too hot in bed - Stuffy, airless surroundings - After a warm bath	- Rest - Lying down - Being in a moderately warm room	**Sulphur**

vaginal dryness

This problem is a common feature of menopausal changes and can be attributed to declining levels of the female sex hormone oestrogen that is responsible for the skin becoming drier, thinner and more prone to signs of ageing.

Rather grim as this sounds, it is important to note that while these changes are fairly common once menopause is well under way, they are by no means inevitably severe. More importantly, if vaginal dryness does show signs of becoming a problem, there is a great deal of complementary and conventional medical help and advice that can improve the situation.

Common symptoms of vaginal dryness can include any of the following:

- **Increased susceptibility to vaginal and urinary tract infections due to there being less natural protection as oestrogen levels decline**
- **Pain and discomfort during sex, which can lead to a less than enthusiastic sex life.**
- **A thinning of the walls of the vagina can lead to small amounts of spotting and breakthrough bleeding on occasion**

If any of these symptoms are an increasing problem, don't feel you have to put up with it. Either follow the advice listed below or consult a trained homeopathic practitioner who can go far beyond what the self-prescriber is able to achieve.

The answer from a conventional medical perspective is either to apply a local preparation of oestrogen cream or to start hormone replacement therapy. The topical application should plump up the tissues and provide a little more moisture, although the effect will be quite limited. However, owing to concerns regarding the safety of HRT, it makes sense to opt for the plant-based phyto-oestrogen creams as a first resort.

In extreme cases, vaginal dryness can result in a prolapse of the womb which feels like a bearing down sensation that is aggravated by standing for long periods of time or straining to lift heavy objects. It is often accompanied by persistent backache, as well as an urgent and frequent need to pass water, which can be difficult and painful. Pelvic floor exercises can correct a very mild prolapse but surgical intervention will probably be necessary for severe cases.

practical self-help

❧ Regular orgasms are good for maintaining the health of the vagina. By reaching orgasm, a rush of blood flows to the tissues of the vagina and clitoris and protects their suppleness. As soon as this becomes less regular, as a result of a fall in libido from menopausal changes, vaginal tissues can become uncomfortably sensitive, dry and more prone to infection.

If vaginal dryness makes sex quite painful, use a lubricating gel, ideally made from natural ingredients rather than synthetic chemicals.

If you prefer not to use synthetic hormone preparations, you can use a natural alternative made from soya-based ingredients. Phyto-oestrogens (plant-based oestrogens) have similar benefits to the synthetic formulas without having the same potentially negative side-effects.

If vaginal soreness, inflammation and/or irritation have become a regular occurrence, avoid wearing tight clothes or anything that creates a warm, humid environment around the genital area, as this is where micro-organisms can thrive, and always wear natural cotton or silk underwear. Hold up stockings are preferable to tights and, if you really can't do without jeans, make sure that you wear them for a limited time only and spend the rest of the day in loose, airy clothes.

Avoid highly perfumed bath products that can promote irritation and discomfort and never use deodorants on the vaginal area for the same reason.

Use soothing formulas in your bathwater like a dessertspoon of sea salt, a few drops of lavender or chamomile essential oils or a ready-mixed tincture of Calendula and Hypericum.

A small amount of vitamin E oil applied to the sensitive area in the vagina can ease discomfort and soreness, while encouraging cracked areas to heal.

CAUTION!
• If spotting or intermittent bleeding is present after menopause, seek a medical opinion

TYPE OF VAGINAL DRYNESS	GENERAL SYMPTOMS	WORSE FROM	BETTER FOR	REMEDY NAME
Dryness and intense soreness that is aggravated by movement	- Vaginal dryness may indicate a general lack of moisture in the mucus membranes due to low-grade dehydration - This can also lead to constipation and urinary infections, that trigger a burning sensation in the urethra when passing water	- Moving even slightly - First movement after resting - Becoming overheated	- Coolness, locally applied - Rest - Keeping in one position for as long as possible	**Bryonia**
Vaginal dryness that sets in as a result of a hysterectomy	- Excruciatingly sensitive in areas of the vagina with stinging pains and/or maddening itching - Overall discomfort is much more noticeable when sitting down	- During or after sex - Emotional stress and tension - Touch	- Rest - Warmth	**Staphysagria**
Vaginal dryness with a complete loss of libido	- Severe itching and irritation that is much more noticeable when walking - General sense of uneasiness and discomfort in the vagina may be made more intense by a prolapsed womb (this feels like a bearing down sensation with persistent backache) - Leaking or dribbling of urine can also occur, especially when coughing and/or sneezing	- Touch - Sex - Feeling under emotional strain or pressure	- Vigorous exercise in the open air - Firm pressure - Rest	**Sepia**
Vaginal dryness with a tendency to very dry and sensitive skin	- Strong aversion to sex because of the degree of pain - Burning and smarting sensations in vagina - General picture of discomfort may be aggravated by a prolapse causing backache	- Emotional pressure - Exertion - Displays of physical affection and sympathy - Touch	- Fresh, open air - Cool bathing - Rest - Relaxing breathing	**Natrum mur**

prostate problems

The prostate is a relatively small gland that's positioned around the urethra in men and has a tendency to enlarge with age. Because of this, problems with urination and a general sense of discomfort commonly emerge from middle age onwards – it's been estimated that some degree of prostate enlargement will be present in around 60 per cent of men by the age of sixty, 70 per cent ten years later and so on. Common symptoms of benign prostate enlargement can include any combination of the following in varying degrees of severity:

- **Straining to pass water which flows in a feeble or interrupted stream**
- **Delay at the beginning of the flow of urine**
- **Urinary dribbling or incontinence**
- **A sense that some urine has been left in the bladder after urination**
- **Discomfort on urination**
- **Urinating more frequently, especially overnight**
- **An urgent need to pass water**

If acute complications occur, such as an infection or inflammation of the prostate gland (prostatitis), the following symptoms can develop:

- **A general sense of being under par and ill**
- **Pain and discomfort in the genitals, thighs, and lower back**
- **Pain when ejaculating**
- **Aching that focuses specifically on the region between the scrotum and the anus, or between the thighs and genitals**
- **Discharge from the urethra after intercourse**

Conventional treatment for prostatitis involves the prescription of antibiotics, while management of an enlarged prostrate usually calls for screening procedures in order to rule out the presence of a malignant tumour. Moderate symptoms of benign enlargement may be treated either with drugs that have an antispasmodic effect or ones that relax the muscle fibres in the prostate and urethra. An enlarged prostate indicates a chronic condition and therefore this is not a situation that can be adequately handled by self-help measures alone. It will require a professional assessment but the following advice will provide extremely helpful support to the conventional treatment.

practical self-help

❧ Research has linked a diet that is high in saturated fat with a high risk of prostate cancer and therefore it is a good idea to avoid foods like red meat, creamy salad dressings, mayonnaise and butter. On the other hand, foods that are rich in essential fatty acids like linseeds, walnuts, sunflower and pumpkin seeds, have a beneficial effect on the prostate and it is recommended that you take at least 30g a day.

❧ Increase your intake of both zinc and fibre. Zinc plays a positive role in regulating the sensitivity of prostate cells to sex hormones, significant as enlargement may partly be triggered by the decline in male sex hormones, while fibre assists the absorption of excess male hormones that are excreted through bile in the digestive tract.

❧ Increase your daily intake of antioxidant nutrients as these play a vital role in helping to combat the negative effects of free radical activity in the body and are your best allies in preventing cancer, heart and circulatory disease. To maximise your exposure to antioxidants through diet, eat liberal and frequent portions of red, yellow, orange, dark green and dark purple fruit, berries and vegetables every day.

❧ Herbal formulations that include saw palmetto and Urtica doica can be very effective in reducing the frequency and severity of symptoms associated with benign enlargement of the prostate gland.

❧ Exercise that encourages a more efficient circulation is also good for easing prostate problems. Ideal forms of movement to consider include walking at a brisk pace in the open air, or yoga.

❧ Cut down, or eliminate, from the diet drinks such as tea, coffee and alcohol that increase the possibility of inflammation in the urinary tract.

❧ Certain ingredients common to Far Eastern cuisine, such as soy, rice, Chinese leaves and kohlrabi provide weak plant hormones that can interact favourably with natural male hormones and prevent prostate complications.

CAUTION!

IF ANY OF THE FOLLOWING OCCUR, CONSULT YOUR DOCTOR:

- Pronounced weight loss
- Traces of blood in urine or semen
- Tiredness for no apparent reason
- Reduced appetite
- Pains in the bones
- Anaemia
- Pain on ejaculation

TYPE OF PROSTATE PROBLEM	GENERAL SYMPTOMS	WORSE FROM	BETTER FOR	REMEDY NAME
Benign enlargement with thin stream of urine that takes a while to get going	- Irritating sensation as though a drop of urine is left in the urethra after passing water - Burning sensation between urinating - Frequent need to urinate; may be passed very slowly	- After sex - Touch - After passing water - Invasive screening and surgery	- Warmth locally applied - Resting	**Staphysagria**
Enlarged prostate with dribbling of urine when stressed	- Urination is slow to start and requires a lot of straining in order to achieve a satisfactory flow and pressure - Murky look to urine with deposits that look like sand or gravel - Travelling makes frequency and urgency more intense	- Anxiety and stress - On waking from sleep - Becoming overheated - Pressure of tight clothes	- Coolness locally applied - When urinating - Mental distraction and absorption - Gentle exercise	**Lycopodium**
Prostate problems that are more problematic when resting	- Discomfort and urinary incontinence are more noticeable in bed at night - Regularly interrupted flow with urine stopping and starting fitfully - Constant urge to pass water when lying down	- During the night - After eating - Too much fatty food - Becoming hot and stuffy	- Standing up - Contact with fresh air - Gentle exercise that doesn't overheat	**Pulsatilla**
Inflamed prostate with pains that radiate down the thighs	- Involuntary dribbling of urine when coughing or sneezing - Pains may be worse on, or completely restricted to, the right side - Spasmodic pains on attempting to pass urine	- Excessive stress - Cold draughts - Coffee - Alcohol - Lack of exercise	- After a sound sleep - Peace and quiet - Lying on one side	**Nux vomica**

homeopathy

●

changes in libido

Approaching middle age can be a source of great trepidation for all sorts of reasons, such as a changing sense of identity, fearing the signs of ageing and being uneasy about losing one's competitive edge and va-va-voom. However, there is one particular issue that is often central to any anxiety about getting older and this is fear of the signs of a flagging or absent libido.

While it is only natural, as you get older, to expect changes in the pace and nature of a sexual encounter, this doesn't mean that you have to say goodbye to an active and satisfying sex life. Even allowing for the physical changes that women especially notice at this time, many couples see this period as an opportunity that allows them new and precious freedoms.

Once menopause has been achieved, liberation from the need for contraception can lead to a much more spontaneous sex life, as can the freedom from interruption when young children have begun to lead independent lives of their own. Mid-life can also be a positive phase when emotional and sexual confidence has moved on in line with life experience, and you can be much more articulate and honest about emotional and sexual needs and preferences.

These are some of the real advantages and yet, of course, it would be inaccurate not to mention some of the disadvantages that can accompany mid-life and especially those that have a negative effect on the libido. These can include any of the following:

- **Relationship problems**
- **Lack of effective communication**
- **Poor self-esteem and self-confidence**
- **Depression**
- **Fatigue, boredom or lack of motivation**
- **Painful intercourse**

Bear in mind that some conventional drugs can be responsible for a lowered libido, particularly those prescribed for high blood pressure, depression and allergies. If you would like to know more about this, consult your pharmacist or family doctor about any medication you are taking.

A conventional medical approach will want to rule out other causes, such as peri-menopausal or menopausal symptoms, thyroid imbalance, or prostate problems. It should also explore any underlying issues that can contribute to a flagging libido, and may suggest counselling for stress management, relationship problems or depression. Hormone replacement therapy may be suggested for both men and women but this form of treatment is quite controversial, as there is no hard and fast research evidence to prove this can restore a flagging libido.

practical self-help

❧ If relationship issues are getting in the way of a fulfilling sex life, it may be helpful to seek counselling in order to clear the air in an emotionally safe environment. Problems and tensions often arise at mid-life that can impact negatively on self-esteem and as both male and female partners are likely to be grappling with these issues at the same time, it can be very constructive to talk them through with a trained listener.

❧ Specific physical sexual problems may benefit from the help of a sex therapist, who will be able to give advice on dealing with common symptoms that can inhibit sexual activity, such as premature ejaculation, difficulty maintaining an erection and vaginal soreness.

❧ When energy levels are low, a diminishing libido is usually the first sign that all is not well. If you suddenly fancy a cup or tea or a glass of gin more than a passionate encounter, consider if your energy levels have been going adrift and, if this is the case, see the 'Tired all the Time' section on page 70 of chapter three.

❧ Boredom can inevitably sneak in quietly at the back door of long-term relationships. Try introducing some fresh passion into the bedroom by taking time for each other and talking about your needs and desires. Make the bedroom warm, perfumed and softly lit and choose times of the day or night that best suit you and your energy levels.

❧ Specific foods and spices are thought to act as natural aphrodisiacs. These include asparagus, shellfish, herrings, wholegrains, nuts, seeds, celery, parsnip, ginger and cinnamon. Also bear in mind that alcohol acts as a depressant so try to avoid it as much as possible.

❧ Ylang ylang is a very sensual essential oil, as well as having mood-balancing properties. As a result, it's ideal for vaporising in the bedroom and/or adding to bathwater.

TYPE OF FLAGGING LIBIDO	GENERAL SYMPTOMS	WORSE FROM	BETTER FOR	REMEDY NAME
Loss of libido as a result of extreme exhaustion	- Apathetic and indifferent to the whole idea of sex following a period of very high stress - General sense of being mentally and physically drained - The whole genital area feels weak	- Sexual activity - Emotional pressure - Cold	- Having a nap - Resting - Warmth	**Phos ac**
Withdrawn, sluggish and miserable with no libido	- Libido has disappeared as a result of depression and/or physical discomfort of having sex - Vagina feels hot and dry with thin discharge - Ejaculation happens prematurely	- Exertion and physical effort - Becoming cold - At night	- Being touched - After moderate exercise in the fresh air - Eating	**Graphites**
Loss of libido after invasive tests to the genital area	- If examinations have been painful or invasive, a memory of violation can make intimacy difficult - The genital area may feel painfully sensitive with stinging, sharp pains on being touched	- Emotional upset - Touch - Attempting sexual intercourse	- Rest - Warmth	**Staphysagria**
Loss of libido from menopausal depression	- Mentally, emotionally and physically drained; feels stretched to the limit with sex feeling like yet another pressure - Indifferent and/or irritable to sexual partner	- Leading up to or following the menopause - Sitting still - After sex - Emotional responsibilities	- After a good night's sleep - Fresh air - Aerobic exercise	**Sepia**
Loss of libido from lack of confidence	- Feelings of insecurity often find expression in aggression and sarcasm - Prostate problems can lead to weak erections which make self-esteem issues worse - Sex is uncomfortable due to a burning sensation in the vagina during or after intercourse	- Stress - On waking - After eating - Thinking about future pressures that need to be met	- Mental distraction - Gentle exercise - Stable temperatures	**Lycopodium**

weight gain

This is not an issue that's confined to mid-life but there are various reasons why concerns about carrying extra weight become a more pressing issue as the years accumulate. These can be linked to the following factors:

- **Lack of regular exercise**
- **Comfort eating due to emotional issues such as fear of ageing, the need to find a new identity and role and pressures that may come from caring for ageing relatives**
- **The natural slowing down process that undoubtedly impacts on your metabolic rate as you get older**

The whole issue of dieting is a very controversial one, as, on its own, it really isn't an adequate tool for keeping weight off over time. Diets may help you shed excess pounds but it is very unlikely that they will stay off forever; you are almost guaranteed to put it all back on again once your lifestyle has returned to normal.

Complementary medicine, sadly, can't wave a magic wand to make those unwanted pounds disappear but holistic therapies such as homeopathy have a great deal to offer by aiming to get your whole system working at its optimum efficiency. Furthermore, if you match this with positive lifestyle changes, then it is far easier to regulate your weight over the long-term. The advice that follows may be enough to get you moving in a positive direction but for more resistant, well-established problems with weight gain or eating issues, it is a good idea to consult an experienced homeopathic practitioner.

practical self-help

❧ If you feel that your system has become sluggish and it takes far less food to put on the pounds than it did a few years ago, this can probably be explained by the natural slowing down of metabolic rate from mid-life onwards. One of the most effective ways of tackling this situation is to take regular exercise three or four times a week. (Research suggests that it is far more important to do three or four forty-minute sessions a week rather than going hell for leather at a two-hour session once a fortnight.) As long as this routine is kept up, the benefits, in terms of a more efficient metabolic rate, will continue. However, unfortunately, as soon as you stop, the metabolism will revert to its slower cruising level and so it is very important that you choose a form of exercise that you will enjoy, and one that is appropriate to your level of fitness.

❧ Calculate precisely how much you eat over a period of twenty-four hours. The only way to do this accurately is to write down every item of food and drink that passes your lips. If you do this for a week or so you'll probably be surprised at the amount you consume, and also how it differs from what you remember. However, it will provide you with a realistic base from which to make healthy adjustments.

❧ Avoid yo-yo dieting as it impacts negatively on your metabolic rate over the long term, while increasing your susceptibility to cellulite and stretch marks. Instead, make realistic improvements to your food intake, concentrating on items that are naturally high in fibre, low in saturated fat and white sugar and that provide you with healthy amounts of protein. This combination will give you everything to build, repair and maintain healthy cells in your body and will also keep your blood sugar levels as stable as possible so you won't get ravenously hungry. Items to avoid at all costs are fairly obvious and include anything made from white, refined, sugar that is full of empty calories (i.e. with no nutritional benefits). Don't forget to eliminate hidden sources of white sugar, such as in ketchups, sweet tomato sauces, baked beans and processed savoury foods like pizzas. In addition, steer clear of snacks that contain a hefty amount of unhealthy, transfatty acids, such as heavily emulsified, processed cheeses, crisps, cakes and puddings. These not only encourage the production of free radicals in the body but also adversely effect the hormonal balance; they boost prostaglandin production to an unhealthy degree, giving rise to symptoms that resemble PMS such as fluid retention and mood swings.

❧ Don't be fooled into thinking that 'low cal' versions of processed foods and drinks must be a healthy option. In fact, the reverse is probably true for, if you examine the label, you are likely to see a significant number of artificial sweeteners and other chemical flavourings. Research from the United States suggests that a regular intake of artifical sweeteners can disrupt the body's natural ability to assess the calorific value of food by its sweetness. As a result, you can end up craving more and more sweet foods, rather than re-educating your taste buds towards healthy, more natural alternatives.

CAUTION!

If you consistently put on weight for no good reason and this is combined with marked fatigue, dry skin, constipation and low moods, go and see your doctor who can check the health of your thyroid gland

TYPE OF WEIGHT PROBLEM	GENERAL SYMPTOMS	WORSE FROM	BETTER FOR	REMEDY NAME
Weight gain with a general feeling that the whole system has become sluggish	- Weight gain is combined with tiredness, a disinclination to engage in any form of exercise, and an overall sense of flabbiness - Digestion happens slowly with a tendency to indigestion and constipation - Flushes readily on exertion	- Becoming chilled - Mental or physical effort - Tight clothes - At menopause	- Dry, warm weather - Resting - Massage	**Calc carb**
Weight gain with cravings for salty, savoury and fatty foods	- Comfort eating as a result of emotional stress or trauma can lead to putting on extra pounds - Instead of talking and working through emotions, feelings are turned inward and suppressed	- Emotional outbursts - Sympathy - Stodgy, fatty or salty foods - Being hugged	- Contact with fresh air - Resting - Skipping meals	**Natrum mur**
Weight gain from acquiring a taste for junk foods	- This remedy can help break an addictive cycle involving coffee, chocolate, alcohol and sugar, which may have developed as a result of high stress levels and a corresponding need to comfort eat	- High levels of stress and pressure - First thing in the morning - Lack of sound, refreshing sleep	- Peace and quiet - Release or management of stress	**Nux vomica**
Weight gain with a craving for sweet things	- Appetite can become disordered with a tendency to snack on sweets rather than eat at proper meal times - Wakes in the night feeling ravenously hungry and has to get up and eat	- Waking from sleep - After eating - Mid-afternoon - Indigestible foods	- Warm drinks - Loosening clothes - Burping	**Lycopodium**

mid-life crises

There are a number of very good reasons why approaching mid-life can feel like a bit of an emotional minefield, and they can include any of the following:

- **Fear of the ageing process and the physical and mental changes that are associated with it**
- **Questioning your identity at the prospect of retirement, children growing up and leaving home, the break up of a long-term relationship or just a general feeling of 'is this really it?'**
- **Fear of death**
- **Bereavement**
- **Panic about losing sexual desirability and potency**

Alarming as these issues can undoubtedly be, it is helpful to bear in mind that whatever form your particular mid-life crisis may take (and you never know, you may not have one), it can be a catalyst for positive change and help you move forward as a stronger and ultimately more confident person. Common symptoms can include any of the following problems:

- **Mood swings**
- **Irritability, tearfulness and/or jitteriness**
- **Poor sleep pattern**
- **Anxiety and/or depression**
- **Irregularities in appetite with loss of pleasure in eating and/or bouts of comfort eating**
- **Lack of mental focus and concentration**
- **Tension headaches**
- **Muscular aches and pains**
- **Palpitations (awareness of a fluttering or fast heartbeat)**

It would be foolish to suggest that complementary medicine is able to sort out symptoms of mid-life crises at a stroke and yet it can provide a very important support through the whole process of transition. If symptoms are severe, or refuse to respond to self-help measures alone, you will need to consult a trained practitioner, especially if at any time you suffer from prolonged periods of anxiety and depression.

practical self-help

❧ If you are finding it hard to leave a younger identity behind, such as being a mother with children at home, it may help to retrain and start a fresh career. It is not at all uncommon for a new role in life to emerge from mid-life onwards and this often provides a renewed sense of excitement, achievement and direction in life. Check with your local colleges to see what courses interest you, talk to voluntary organisations who need extra help or even start up your own small business.

❧ Low self-esteem and anxiety may respond favourably to Cognitive Behavioural Therapy, which enables the client to identify negative thought patterns that have developed since childhood and find more positive ways of confronting situations that are causing distress.

❧ Relationship problems can often be better understood, and even resolved, with the help of a specialist counselor and, when the relationship has ended, talking to a professional can also enable you to move on and remain positive.

❧ If low-grade anxiety and wobbly confidence are a problem, taking a few drops of Rescue Remedy is a fast-acting, practical aid for when tension levels are high. Either dissolve a drop directly under the tongue or dilute a few drops in a glass of water and sip at intervals. (It is safe to take with conventional medication and/or homeopathic remedies.)

❧ Symptoms of mild to moderate depression may emerge at mid-life for any of the reasons mentioned above. If this is the case, consider taking a course of St John's Wort for gentle emotional support without any of the side effects that accompany many anti-depressants. St John's Wort does however interact with a few conventional drugs such as some contraceptive pills, limited types of asthma medication and some of the drugs that are used to prevent the body rejecting an organ transplant. Therefore, if you are in any doubt about its suitability in your case, don't self-medicate but consult your pharmacist or doctor.

CAUTION!

IF ANY OF THE FOLLOWING OCCUR, SEEK PROMPT MEDICAL ADVICE:

- **Severe mood swings**
- **Lack of motivation to the point of avoiding professional and domestic tasks**
- **Seriously disrupted sleep pattern that refuses to sort itself out**
- **A sense of emotional numbness, unreality or being permanently distanced from others**

Homeopathic Support Table overleaf

TYPE OF MID-LIFE CRISIS	GENERAL SYMPTOMS	WORSE FROM	BETTER FOR	REMEDY NAME
Fear of death as the ultimate expression of a loss of control	- Anxiety is especially severe at night, with a tendency to wake from sleep around 2a.m. feeling sick and fearful - Phobias may develop around illness as a result of feeling tense and anxious - Restlessness is eased by getting up and having a warm drink	- After midnight - Feeling cold and chilled - Alcohol - Smoking	- Warmth - Lying with the head higher than the body - Company - Movement	**Arsenicum album**
Loss of sexual confidence as a result of low-grade depression	- Feeling flat takes all the zest out of life, including motivation for relationships and work - Because of diminished mental, emotional and physical energy, sex becomes just another demand to be met	- During the menopause - Waking from sleep - After sex - Being touched - Domestic chores	- Aerobic exercise in the fresh air - Warmth - Stimulating company	**Sepia**
Bouts of severe weepiness that are connected to a profound sense of loss	- Grieving lost youth or feeling acute separation anxiety as children leave home - Moods change rapidly from feeling cheerful to sadness and grief - Sighs involuntarily and feels as though there's a constant lump of emotion in the throat	- Emotional strain - Sense of loss - Coffee - Smoking - Making a physical effort	- When alone - Breathing deeply - Eating small amounts - Warmth	**Ignatia**
Low mood that descends as a result of anger turned inwards	- Pent-up anger about a major issue festers and comes out as a disproportionate rage over trifling issues, or as a low, sad, extra-sensitive mood	- Emotional outbursts - Anger - Sexual release - At night	- Resting - Warmth	**Staphysagria**
Loss of confidence when faced with change	- Vulnerability takes refuge in a critical, bossy manner - Physical changes at mid-life can provoke anxiety about sexual inadequacies	- On waking from sleep - After eating - Pressure	- Moderate exercise in the fresh air - Urination	**Lycopodium**

circulatory problems
(chilblains and reynaud's syndrome)

Increasing age isn't the only reason for circulatory disorders, it's just that these problems have a tendency to become proportionally more common with the passage of time. Chilblains occur in cold weather as a result of poor circulation to the hands and feet; the skin often turns a bluish-purple and an itch-scratch-itch cycle can be set off if the affected areas become heated very quickly.

Reynaud's Syndrome is triggered by the small blood vessels that supply the fingers and toes when they become hypersensitive to the cold. The affected areas turn white and experience a tingling, pain and/or burning sensations before they return to a normal colour. Conventional treatments focus on the application of topical creams in order to soothe the pain and discomfort of chilblains and the prescription of drugs that aim to relax and open the blood vessels for the treatment of Reynaud's Syndrome.

practical self-help

- During the autumn and winter months always keep exposed areas like fingers and ears well covered and wrapped up, and always wear a warm pair of socks.
- When thawing out after exposure to cold winds, always avoid the temptation to roast the hands or feet close to a fire or heater as this can trigger a bout of itching. Instead, thaw cold fingers and toes out gently and slowly under warm running water.
- Increase the efficiency of your circulation by taking regular, rhythmic exercise that stimulates the heart and lungs.
- Gently massage the hands and feet each night, regardless of the season, in order to stimulate and encourage efficient circulation in these areas.
- Include wheatgerm products and unroasted, unsalted nuts in your diet, as these are naturally rich sources of vitamin E, which prevents blood clots from forming in the arteries, enhances the red blood cells' capacity to transport oxygen and dilates the capillaries.
- Gently rub soothing tamus cream onto chilblains that are cracked and painful.
- If the skin around the affected area isn't cracked, two drops of lavender and two drops of tea tree essential oils can be added to a teaspoon of carrier oil and gently massaged in to relieve pain and inflammation.

CAUTION!

The situation should be checked out if symptoms of Reynaud's or chilblains are combined with episodes of breathlessness, fatigue and/or chest pains on exertion

Homeopathic Support Table overleaf

TYPE OF CIRCULATORY PROBLEM	GENERAL SYMPTOMS	WORSE FROM	BETTER FOR	REMEDY NAME
Burning, itching skin that is very sensitive to cold air	- Itchy, sensitive skin that becomes dry and thickened after exposure to cold - Feet and legs feel achy as a result of poor circulation - Warm bathing is soothing to areas that feel uncomfortable	- Undressing - Cold draughts of air - Sweating - Contact with damp	- Gentle rubbing rather than scratching - Warm, dry conditions	**Rhus tox**
Maddeningly itchy chilblains	- Burning areas of skin that feel swollen and look red; once one patch is scratched, itching moves to a fresh area - Skin bruises readily after minor trauma	- Contact with cold, sharp winds - Touch	- Keeping the limbs moving	**Agaricus**
Chapped, cracked skin on fingers and toes after exposure to cold winds	- The tips of the fingers split very easily in very cold conditions - Fingers and toes take on a purple-looking tinge, with a tendency to develop chilblains that burn and itch	- Touch or pressure of clothing - During the winter months	- Dry, warm weather	**Petroleum**
Burning, itching sensations in the extremeties react badly to heat	- Although very chilly, exposure to stuffy, overheated rooms feels uncomfortable - Poor circulation in the hands and feet makes them feel permanently cold and yet the feet can also experience a burning sensation in bed at night - Symptoms often set in when you become chilled after being too hot	- Becoming overheated - Stuffy rooms - In bed at night	- Gentle exercise - Contact with fresh air - Taking clothes off	**Pulsatilla**

fatigue

See 'Tired all the Time' in chapter three on page 70 as the advice in this section is as relevant to lagging energy levels at mid-life as it is at any other time of life. In addition, consider having a blood test in order to check that specific conditions, such as anaemia, irregular thyroid function and Type 2 (maturity onset) diabetes aren't complicating the situation.

high blood pressure

High blood pressure does not manifest any symptoms and therefore it is one of those tricky medical conditions that often goes unnoticed until you have a routine medical examination. However, it is very important to have regular check-ups as blood pressure readings can be important indicators of circulatory, kidney, and heart disease. The conventional treatment for high blood pressure focuses on lifestyle advice and also, possibly, prescription drugs.

High blood pressure is a chronic condition and therefore, if symptoms have reached a severe or established stage, you should seek assessment and treatment from a trained homeopathic practitioner. However, the following advice will be extremely useful for anyone who has borderline high blood pressure and wants to see if acute homeopathic intervention can help bring it down to a more acceptable level.

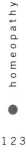
practical self-help

☙ Check the amount of salt you take on a daily basis, being especially aware of convenience foods, take-away dishes and even some forms of mineral water.

☙ Take time out each day to relax as one of the main features of the stress response includes raised blood pressure. Meditation, for example, encourages the relaxing branch of the autonomic nervous system to kick in and counteract the opposite side, which is fired when you are under stress.

☙ Don't drink more than two cups of coffee a day or three cups of tea a day as caffeine stimulates the secretion of stress hormones that, in turn, raise blood pressure that can remain elevated on a long-term basis.

☙ Take gentle, regular areobic exercise as it burns off excess adrenalin, while also encouraging the secretion of natural, feel-good chemicals called endorphins.

☙ If you are a smoker, the single most important thing you can do is give it up. Smoking is associated with a whole host of health problems; including furred-up arteries, raised high blood pressure and an increased risk of heart disease.

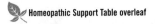 Homeopathic Support Table overleaf

TYPE OF BLOOD PRESSURE	GENERAL SYMPTOMS	WORSE FROM	BETTER FOR	REMEDY NAME
High blood pressure with cravings for salt and fat	- Apart from dietary factors, cruising blood pressure readings can be raised by a tendency to suppressed emotions - Fluid retention may also be noticeable	- Emotional stress or trauma - Becoming overheated - Sympathy or attention	- Gentle exercise - Fresh, open air - Cool bathing	**Natrum mur**
High blood pressure as a result of too much caffeine and junk food	- When high blood pressure is the result of eating and drinking unwisely over the years and also compounded with lots of stress, it can be very difficult to switch off successfully and relax	- Coffee - Alcohol - Lack of sleep - On waking	- Resting - Sound, undisturbed sleep - As the day goes on	**Nux vomica**
High blood pressure from unexpressed anger	- Very short-fused and inclined to fly off the handle for the most trivial reasons - Trembling and palpitations make it very difficult to switch off and go to sleep	- Becoming irritated - Smoking - Mental effort or strain - Being touched	- After eating - Rest - Warmth	**Staphysagria**

CAUTION!

High blood pressure that refuses to come down in response to self-help measures or complementary medical treatment will need attention and treatment from your doctor

osteoarthritis

The arthritic aches and pains that are generally associated with the wear and tear effect of getting older, will most often be due to osteoarthritis. Every joint in the body is cushioned with a layer of cartilage and, over the years, this gets worn, distorted or thickens with daily use; it can sometimes feel as if the bones that make up a joint are grinding against each other. This condition causes swelling and stiffness in the large, weight-bearing joints of the hips, and knees, and the severity and frequency of the pain varies according to weather conditions; cold and damp can be especially difficult for some sufferers. Movement can ease or noticeably aggravate pain depending on the individual.

Conventional treatment initially focuses on ways of managing the pain through painkillers and anti-inflammatories but surgery may be considered if the joint has become unusable through pain and stiffness. This would involve a joint replacement which, when done successfully, can restore a full range of movement that is free from pain.

The following advice will help for the odd twinge and also for pains that are already frequent and severe as it can be used in a supporting role with your conventional treatment.

practical self-help

❧ A combined glucosamine and condroitin supplement can be a very effective, natural anti-inflammatory formula that noticeably reduces pain and stiffness in the joints. You can buy it in tablet form but, if you are already taking prescription drugs, check with your pharmacist that it is appropriate, before you self-medicate.

❧ Avoid red meat, foods or drinks that include a high proportion of refined, white sugar, dairy products, nightshade-type vegetables (aubergines, tomatoes and peppers) and citrus fruit. If you suspect one of these might be causing or aggravating problems, drop it from your diet for a month and assess how you feel when you re-introduce it again. If symptoms flare up, cut the suspect item out again for another four weeks before introducing it once more. If there is another adverse reaction then you are probably better off without it.

❧ If joint pain and stiffness are much more noticeable in cold, wet weather and feel considerably eased by limbering up through gentle exercise, try rubbing Rhus tox cream into the affected areas after a long soak in a warm bath.

❧ Joint pain and stiffness that responds well to contact with cool air will do better with glucosamine gel, taken straight from the fridge and applied to the affected areas.

❧ It's essential to keep joints as mobile as possible as otherwise stiffness and lack of flexibility can become a real problem. However, it is best to avoid any activity that puts strain on the joints through repetitive, jarring movements on hard surfaces.

Homeopathic Support Table overleaf

TYPE OF ARTHRITIC PAIN	GENERAL SYMPTOMS	WORSE FROM	BETTER FOR	REMEDY NAME
Joint pains that date from a fall or injury	- Joints and surrounding muscles feel stiff, bruised and aching - Stiffness and pains in hip joints can trigger a feeling of weakness and wobbliness when walking	- Jarring - Touch - Physical effort - Pressure	- Resting in a comfortable position	**Arnica**
Pain in joints with cold, numb sensation	- Pains move in an upward direction from the ankles and feet to the hips - This remedy can relieve the afterpains of a steroid injection, provided the symptoms fit	- Becoming warm or warmth locally applied - Alcohol - Moving - During the night	- Bathing the stiff, painful area with cool water - Resting	**Ledum**
Stiff, painful joints that look pale red and swollen	- Joints feel hot with severe tearing pains that cause great restlessness - Even the slightest movement increases the pain and distress - The system feels generally toxic with joint pains	- Even the slightest movement - Stooping - Sudden, jarring movements like coughing - Light touch	- Resting and keeping still in one position - Firm pressure - Lying on the painful limb	**Bryonia**
Stiff, painful joints that are always more of a problem in winter	- Joint pains are especially severe in bed at night, causing uncomfortable restlessness - Pain and stiffness are especially noticeable first thing in the morning and get easier as they limber up during the day	- Cold, damp weather - Resting - During the night - Jolting	- Gentle exercise for a limited period of time - Warmth - Massage - Support to the affected area	**Rhus tox**
Painful, swollen joints that look puffy, pale pink and water-logged	- Severe stinging pains in arthritic joints that flare up quickly and dramatically - Prickly pains and swelling may especially affect the ankle joints - Swollen skin has a tendency to 'pit' when light pressure is applied	- Becoming overheated - Contact with warmth in any form - Rest - After sleep	- Contact with anything cool - Gentle movement - Taking clothes off	**Apis**

homeopathy
for cosmetic problems

6

With so many recent advances in skincare for treating specific problem areas, it is not surprising that many people assume it is what is applied to the skin that is most important in correcting cosmetic problems. However, while there are obvious benefits to using products that make the skin feel softer and look clearer, the homeopathic approach is able to take treatment beyond the superficial and restore the imbalance that lies deeper in the body's constitution.

For example, a tendency to eczema is thought to be a symptom of the body's generalised hypersensitivity that can also be linked to hay fever and/or asthma. Therefore, homeopathic treatments, in common with a range of other popular complementary therapies such as traditional Chinese medicine and western medical herbalism, will treat this cosmetic problem from within, rather than simply aiming to keep the symptoms temporarily at bay with a cream or lotion. When the correct remedy is prescribed, they should clear up altogether, or at least become so mild or infrequent that they are, at most, a very minor nuisance.

eczema

With infantile eczema, the most susceptible areas tend to be the flexions inside the forearm and behind the knee but they can also be any place where the body is particularly warm and where there is a skin fold; behind the ears, under the breasts and around the eyelids. Although the severity and pattern of distribution varies immensely, any combination of the following can be regarded as a common feature of eczema:

- **Red, itchy patches of skin that may, or may not be raised**
- **Clusters of intensely itchy blisters that dry out to form a crusty surface after scratching**
- **Bleeding or weeping of the skin as a result of constant itching**
- **Soreness and burning of the affected areas**
- **Stinging pain in raw areas**

The conventional medical approach most commonly prescribes steroid creams for sore, itchy areas. In cases where a secondary infection has set in as a result of the skin being broken, creams often combine a steroid ingredient with a topical antibiotic. Occasionally, doctors prescribe an oral antihistamine medication in order to calm down widespread itching and discomfort.

It needs to be stressed at this stage that the sort of eczema that can be improved by using the complementary medical strategies listed below must be of the mildest, most minor kind. Anything of a more severe and chronic nature needs to be treated by an experienced homeopath as they will be able to provide the more ambitious, constitutional treatment. Furthermore, there is a risk that taking a remedy too frequently can intensify the symptoms and therefore it is best for a skilled professional to handle this quite volatile skin condition.

practical self-help

❧ Dry and taut skin can be greatly soothed by an oatmeal bath; collect a generous handful of oatmeal in a fine muslin bag and suspend it just below the hot tap as the bathwater runs. Soak in the oatmeal-softened water for as long as feels comfortable.

❧ If strictly controlled exposure to sunlight helps clear your skin, check with your pharmacist that the sun care products you are using are suitable for anyone with even mild eczema. Some contain para-aminobenzoic acid (PABA) to block the damaging effect of UV rays and these can be particularly inflammatory to sensitive skins.

❧ If contact with detergents aggravates your skin, clean with allergy-free products and always rinse the washing twice over. If chopping fruit or vegetables causes a problem, wear thin cotton gloves for protection.

❧ Specific small patches of mildly irritated or dry skin can be soothed and encouraged to heal with a topical application of Calendula cream. However, do a patch test on the inside of your wrist, waiting a couple of days to see if your skin takes it well. If it doesn't sting on application, apply it twice a day to the affected areas after showering or bathing.

❧ Always moisturise after a bath, as they can have a strong dehydrating effect on the skin and dry skin is far more likely to feel itchy and irritated. Experiment with naturally based products that include soothing essential oils such as lavender and chamomile.

CAUTION!

IF ANY OF THE FOLLOWING OCCUR, CONSULT YOUR DOCTOR:

• **Severe inflammation and itching that leads to bleeding and crusting of the affected area**

• **Weeping of the itchy area that may involve secretion of a clear fluid**

• **Eczema that is obviously spreading and/or becoming more severe in nature – medical attention is especially crucial for young babies**

TYPE OF ECZEMA	GENERAL SYMPTOMS	WORSE FROM	BETTER FOR	REMEDY NAME
Localised patches of dry burning skin that are soothed by contact with warmth	- Symptoms may be more noticeable when stress or anxiety levels are high - Affected areas look blistery, and feel very itchy after scratching - Discomfort and restlessness is more noticeable at night and during the early hours of the morning	- Becoming cold or chilled - High levels of stress - Alcohol	- Warm compresses - Letting warm air get to the skin - Being distracted and having company	**Arsenicum album**
Eczema that's especially noticeable in skin folds	- Affected patches feel rough and thicker than other areas - Constant itching makes the skin bleed, which then forms a crust - Skin may show a general tendency to slow healing and fast infection	- In winter - Touching sore areas	- In dry, warm weather	**Petroleum**
Patches of eczema that become crusty quickly	- Skin has a general tendency to become cracked very quickly around the edges of the lips, nose, ears and nipples - Affected areas bleed readily after scratching - Especially well indicated for weepy eczema	- During the night - After scratching - Getting too hot - Leading up to, and after a period	- Exposing sore areas to the fresh air	**Graphites**
Eczema that is part of a tendency for skin to become chapped and dry	- Skin is generally pale, clammy and cool to the touch, with a history of poor healing - Eczema surfaces in childhood or around the menopause - General tendency to sensitive, dry, cracked skin may be complicated by an underfunctioning thyroid gland, leading to weight gain	- Bathing - Contact with raw, cold air - Seasonal change; approaching winter - Drinking milk - High anxiety levels	- Rubbing rather than scratching - Dry, mild weather	**Calc carb**

homeopathy

129

psoriasis

This chronic problem occurs because the skin develops a tendency to turn over cells too rapidly. As a result, thick, dry, scaly patches develop that may be itchy. Elbows, knees and the scalp are all generally affected, with patches often occurring symmetrically in an oval shape. Scaling can be especially problematic on the scalp, with flakes imitating a very severe case of dandruff. In addition, the hair on the crown of the head and around the hairline generates heat while on the face, the eyebrows can look as though they have dandruff and scaly patches appear anywhere on the face and neck. The nails on the hands and feet are inclined to thicken and become brittle and discoloured and often grow away from the nail bed.

Management of psoriasis, from a conventional medical perspective, uses sunlight treatment and/or the topical application of creams, lotions and shampoos that aim to soothe the skin and reduce the flakiness. As with eczema, any of the following measures can be used in the short-term to ease a mild flare-up of psoriasis. However, long-established and/or severe cases will benefit from professional complementary treatment.

practical self-help

❧ Moderate sun exposure can improve many cases of psoriasis but avoid the fierce heat during the middle of the day. Also, check with your pharmacist that the sun protection formula you are using is suitable for psoriasis sufferers.

❧ Foods like red meat, animal fats, white sugar, strong tea, coffee and alcohol put a toxic stress load on the body and can therefore aggravate symptoms of psoriasis.

❧ Oil of evening primrose has an anti-inflammatory effect and studies suggest that this supplement can ease psoriasis symptoms. Unperfumed skin creams containing evening primrose oil can also be helpful in relieving the inflammation and the itching.

❧ Stress is often a major aggravating factor so it is well worth learning practical relaxation techniques such as slow, controlled breathing, yoga, Tai chi and Pilates.

❧ Baths with Dead Sea salts can ease some of the itching and/or inflammation of psoriasis. Try bathing a small area first, two or three times, so as to check how your skin takes it before you immerse your whole body.

CAUTION!

IF ANY OF THE FOLLOWING OCCUR, CONSULT YOUR DOCTOR:

- **Associated joint pains that emerge where psoriasis affects the small joints of the fingers and toes**
- **Signs that patches are spreading to new areas of the body, or existing patches are becoming larger and/or more severe**

TYPE OF PSORIASIS	GENERAL SYMPTOMS	WORSE FROM	BETTER FOR	REMEDY NAME
Burning, dry patches that are briefly soothed by warm bathing	- Skin has a general tendency to become dehydrated and cracked - Psoriasis is likely to be more noticeable and troublesome during, or just after, periods of high anxiety	- Cold in any form - During the night or early hours of the morning	- Soothing, distracting company - Warmth locally applied to irritated patches	**Arsenicum album**
Dry, raw patches that react very badly to warmth	- Symptoms are noticeably more troublesome during, or immediately following, periods of high anticipatory anxiety - Skin on the hands and soles of the feet are especially dry, as well as in the folds - A lot of dandruff-like scaling on the scalp is also common	- Contact with warmth - Tight clothes - Pre-menstrually - Thinking about a coming stressful event	- Gentle movement in the fresh air - Coolness locally applied	**Lycopodium**
Classic psoriasis with thick crusting on the elbows	- Rough, hard, blotchy patches of skin on the elbows with a general tendency to poor circulation - The whole system feels sluggish with a tendency to emotional flatness and physical exhaustion	- Becoming chilled - During or following pregnancy - Scratching	- Warmth locally applied - Getting moving - Aerobic exercise in the fresh air	**Sepia**
Psoriasis that weeps easily after scratching	- Skin is rough and cracked and heals very slowly - Psoriasis patches weep after scratching and this then forms a yellowish crust	- Becoming warm in bed - Becoming chilled - Pre- and post-menstrually - During the night	- Touch - Walking in the fresh air	**Graphites**

cold sores

As with so many other skin conditions, the regular or intermittent appearance of cold sores signifies a deeper-lying problem. In this case, it is the existence of the herpes simplex virus in the system, which can lie dormant for a very long time but which throws up a cold sore at the first sign of developing cold symptoms, of being run down or having too much exposure to sunlight. Symptoms of cold sores vary from one person to another but any combination of the following can be expected:

- **Itching, tingling and/or soreness around the lips, mouth or base of the nostrils**
- **Once a blister forms it is likely to burst and crust over, becoming very hypersenstitive**

Conventional medical approaches tackle the problem by prescribing a topical anti-viral preparation that should be used at the very first twinge or tingle as this heralds the imminent arrival of a cold sore. Any of the following suggestions may be used in combination with conventional treatment and yet, if cold sores are a regular feature of life and/or getting more severe, it is a sign that the body's defence mechanisms are not dealing efficiently with the virus and therefore it would greatly benefit you to consult a homeopathic practitioner.

practical self-help

❧ Apply Rescue Remedy cream as often as feels comfortable to ease the tingling, itching and or soreness.

❧ Apply witch hazel sparingly to the affected area to encourage the cold sore to dry out.

❧ Gently dab the sore area with diluted Hypericum tincture. Add one measure of tincture to ten parts boiled, cooled water and apply on a cotton pad as often as feels soothing.

❧ If a cold sore has surfaced when you feel a bit run down, give your immune system a much-needed boost by taking a course of Echinacea. My recommendation is to take it as an elixir. In order to give the Echinacea the best chance to work, eliminate or cut down on foods and drinks that can compromise the body's immune-system, such as alcohol, coffee and convenience foods.

❧ The virus that triggers cold sores can be carried and transferred on a toothbrush or by oral contact of any kind. Therefore, take preventative action, even if you are in the first stages of twinges and tingling before the blister has actually appeared.

❧ Use a protective sun block when going out in windy, sunny weather, especially if you are near the sea or at high altitude and in the snow, as these conditions magnify the effect of UV light exposure and increase your susceptibility to developing cold sores.

TYPE OF COLD SORE	GENERAL SYMPTOMS	WORSE FROM	BETTER FOR	REMEDY NAME
Cold sores as a result of exposure to sunlight or ongoing emotional stress	- Cold sores often follow a heavy head cold and are most likely to affect the lips, which also have a tendency to dryness and cracking (especially in the middle of the bottom lip) - Affected part of the lip tingles and/or feels numb	- Salty, sea air - Windy, sunny weather - Suppressed emotion and sadness - Touch	- Exposure to cool air - Coolness locally applied	**Natrum mur**
Cold sores that develop above the upper lip	- Sensitive, itching pains in cold sores that bleed very readily - Lips feel and look generally dry, cracked and tight - Skin bruises quickly but tends to heal very slowly	- Salty foods - Any physical contact with the affected area - Cold winds	- Coolness locally and gently applied - Gentle rubbing	**Phosphorus**
Intensely tingly, itchy cold sores that move from the left to the right side of the mouth	- Lips look dry and crack easily in the corners - Cold sores appear on the lips or the area around the mouth - Affected area blisters quickly with strong, numb or crawling sensations where the blister forms	- At night - When resting - Exposure to cold, damp winds - Sudden, jarring movements	- Contact with warm, dry air - Keeping on the move - Warm bathing - Gentle rubbing (taking care not to dislodge the top of the sore)	**Rhus tox**
Cold sores that appear on the mouth, ear lobes and/or corners of the mouth	- If the lower lip is affected, it's likely to feel incredibly swollen and sensitive - The whole system has reached the stage of complete exhaustion - Emotionally at rock bottom with physical discomfort	- Becoming chilled - Pre-menstrually - After pregnancy and childbirth - Rubbing and scratching	- Contact with warmth - Walking or jogging in the fresh air	**Sepia**

homeopathy

133

acne

This troublesome condition has an irritating tendency to surface at times of hormonal upheaval and therefore while most people suffer from teenage acne at one stage of puberty or another, women can unfortunately also break out in spots when they have PMS or go through the menopause. Any of the following symptoms can occur in varying degrees of severity and frequency:

- **Painful, red, 'blind' spots that refuse to come to a head. These often form around the chin and jaw line, sometimes singly but often in tender clusters**
- **Large spots congregate on the oily areas of the forehead, hairline, nose and chin. These often develop a white or yellow head as the heat and pain builds in each individual spot**
- **With established or severe cases, spots spread down the sides of the neck, to the chest and back**
- **Oily skin is generally a sign of overproductive sebaceous glands that block the pores and cause blackheads to form, and yet some dry skins can also be very prone to spots. The latter requires a particularly demanding skin regime as the face is often divided into areas that are oily, and others that are dry and taut. Always use products that are designed for combination skin as anything else will tip the balance and make things worse**

Conventional medical treatments focus on using topical creams and washes to dry mild spots out. In more established or severe cases, drugs may be prescribed to tackle the problem from within and these take the form of a maintenance course of a low-dose antibiotic or a retinoid-type drug that aims to regulate oily secretions.

From a complementary medical perspective, acne is viewed as the tip of an unhealthy iceberg. Therefore, while topical creams are recognised as doing a certain amount of good, the real treatment needs to take place at a deeper level in order to detoxify the system as a whole. This means that positive lifestyle changes can be as important as spending money on lotions and creams that can treat only after the spot has already appeared. When treating spots, think holistically, and you are far more likely to see impressive results, as well as feeling healthier into the bargain. As always, the measures listed opposite are suitable for treating the odd, mild break out of spots. Any situation that's more severe or very well established will demand more long-term treatment from an experienced complementary practitioner.

practical self-help

❧ Drink a healthy amount of water on a daily basis. This helps guard against constipation, which makes the skin more prone to break outs, and also supports the kidneys by flushing them out well. Aim to drink five large glasses of filtered or still mineral water every day and avoid too much tea, coffee and alcohol as these encourage the body to lose fluid and put an extra strain on the liver.

❧ Vitamin C, along with the other antioxidant nutrients vitamin A and E, plays an important role in preserving healthy skin tone and texture. In order to naturally boost your intake through your diet, eat plenty of fresh fruit and vegetables that are bright red, orange, yellow, or dark green in colour. It's slightly harder in the winter months so if you find you are falling short of your five portions a day, take a supplement. Either take vitamin C on its own (500mgs morning and evening), or in an antioxidant combination to support the immune system fight minor infections as well as taking care of your skin.

❧ Certain foods have a reputation for aggravating symptoms of acne and so avoid high-fat items such as cream, full-fat cheese, crisps, chips, roasted and salted nuts and any deep-fried foods that are coated in batter. The latter is especially nasty as it can hold in fat like a sponge.

❧ If you can predict a crop of spots after a period of high stress, incorporate some regular relaxation time into your day and avoid negative behavioural strategies such as relying on alcohol, cigarettes, caffeine and sugar fixes.

❧ Taking radical action to zap away those spots is always very tempting, although bear in mind that desperate measures often backfire. Many acne-targeted face washes are very aggressive and disturb the delicate oil balance of troubled skin, while heavy-duty exfoliators only aggravate sensitivity. As a result, oily patches get oilier and dry patches become unpleasantly taut and flaky. Keep your skin routine as simple and as gentle as possible and only use a clay exfoliator that you can roll off once it has dried. Water-based emulsions are especially suitable for skins that are prone to spots as these provide a light, non-oily lotion that is absorbed quickly and doesn't leave a film behind on the skin.

❧ If spots have left you with scars, apply a tiny amount of vitamin E cream to the affected area to help the skin recover.

❧ Although it's not advisable to overdo facial steaming, moderate amounts can gently and effectively unblock facial pores, especially if you add a drop or two of lavender, bergamot or chamomile essential oil to the steaming water.

homeopathy

135

TYPE OF ACNE	GENERAL SYMPTOMS	WORSE FROM	BETTER FOR	REMEDY NAME
Spots that are very noticeable before a period, during puberty or at the menopause	- Spots move from one area to another, with no two outbreaks seeming the same - Fatty foods trigger the problem or make it more intense - Weepy and emotional about the problem	- Getting too hot - Overly rich foods - Times of hormonal change	- Cooling off - Taking regular, gentle exercise - Coolness locally applied	**Pulsatilla**
Acute and sudden outbreak of bright red spots	- This remedy is most useful in the first 48 hours of the eruption - Spots are large, throbbing and hot - When the remedy works well, it will either calm the spot right down, or move it quickly to the next stage of coming to a head	- Touch or pressure to the sensitive area - Jarring movement - Contact with cold air that chills	- Warmth - Resting	**Belladonna**
Spots that form large, yellow, pus-filled heads	- Skin texture is generally poor and slow to heal, with a tendency to dry, chapped areas as well as oily patches - Throbbing sensation in spots as they come to a head - Great sensitivity to cold draughts	- In the winter - Exposure to dry, cold winds - Touch or pressure	- Humidity - Warmth	**Hepar sulph**
Spots that affect combination skin with a tendency to blocked pores and blackheads	- Although very oily in patches, other parts of the skin crack easily due to chronic dryness - T-zone is often excessively oily while spots on chest and back irritate and feel itchy	- Too much sunlight - Getting too hot - Emotional strain and stress	- Cool water locally applied - Exposing the skin to cool, fresh air	**Natrum mur**
Slow healing skin that tends to scar and/or spots that refuse or are very slow to resolve	- Spots are large and very sensitive and eventually produce a clear, watery pus - Hair and nails may also be in poor condition and break and split easily	- Touch - Humidity - Cold air blowing on the skin	- Warm compresses - Dry, moderately warm weather - During the summer	**Silica**

varicose veins

Although often associated with getting older, varicose veins are by no means a problem that arises only after mid-life as there are many factors that can trigger the condition:

- **A strong inherited tendency**
- **Pregnancy, especially if the baby is large, or if there has been only a short interval of time between pregnancies**
- **Occupational hazards e.g. jobs which involve long periods on your feet, such as hairdressing or working in retail**
- **Wearing hold up stockings that are too tight around the thighs**
- **Being significantly overweight**
- **Suffering from long-term problems with severe constipation**
- **A sedentary lifestyle**

Varicose veins develop when the valves in the veins of the legs are unable to stem the back flow of blood. In time, the veins become knotted and purple and increasingly visible under the surface of the skin. Symptoms vary greatly in their severity, but may include any combination of the following:

- **Throbbing pain and aching in the affected leg(s)**
- **Swelling of the ankles**
- **A general sense of heaviness and discomfort in the legs**
- **Intermittent irritation and itching**

In some cases there is a risk that severe or well-established varicose veins can lead to varicose ulcers, where the skin breaks over the surface of a varicose vein. This is particularly unpleasant as ulcers of this kind can be very stubborn to heal.

Common conventional medical strategies include advice on weight loss, if being significantly overweight is an issue, and resting the feet at the end of the day if swelling is a problem. Treatment for severe varicose veins often involves a course of injections or surgery. The latter removes the troublesome section of vein so that the inefficient valves are left permanently closed. The small, remaining veins then quickly enlarge to take up the slack and transport blood efficiently around the body once more.

Any of the following measures can be used side by side with conventional medical strategies to ease the inflammation, discomfort and swelling of mild to moderate varicose veins. As always, more severe or long-term problems with this condition will require treatment from an experienced homeopathic practitioner and this is especially appropriate if varicose veins are part of a larger picture of circulatory problems.

practical self-help

❧ Avoid standing for extended periods of time as the effect of gravity encourages the blood to 'pool' in the veins of the leg.

❧ Take regular walks as the rhythmical contraction of the muscles in the leg creates a pressure that propels the blood through the valves in the vessels.

❧ Avoid sitting with your legs crossed, as this puts pressure on the veins, and get into the habit of literally putting your feet up in the evening as this will reduce swelling and aching in the congested veins of the legs and ankles.

❧ Take preventative action against chronic constipation as it really isn't worth risking varicose veins in the rectum and/or lining of the anus (called haemorrhoids or piles). The best way to guard against sluggish bowel movements is to drink plenty of water (approximately five large glasses each day) and make naturally high-fibre foods the cornerstone of your diet.

❧ Practise conscious deep breathing techniques as these benefit your circulatory system in general and particularly when combined with regular rhythmical exercise.

❧ Introduce buckwheat into your diet as this is an excellent source of rutin, which has a strengthening effect on the weakened tissue of varicose veins.

❧ The pain and inflammation of varicose ulcers can be soothed by a compress of diluted Calendula tincture (one part tincture to ten parts boiled, cooled water), before applying Calendula cream gently to the affected area.

❧ As long as the skin is unbroken, a compress of witch hazel can give a lot of temporary relief to aching, throbbing varicose veins.

❧ Include lots of grapes, blackcurrants, blueberries, spinach, parsley, citrus fruit, green cabbage and garlic in your diet as these can improve your circulation and help with the gentle elimination of excess fluid from the system.

CAUTION!

IF ANY OF THE FOLLOWING OCCUR, CONSULT YOUR DOCTOR PROMPTLY:

• Persistent and/or very severe pain in a varicose vein

• Marked swelling and aching of the affected leg that isn't promptly eased by raising and resting it

• Accidents that result in the skin over a varicose vein being broken as this can often result in significant blood loss

• Brownish discolouration over any area of the leg where circulation is obviously sluggish and poor

• Ulceration of the skin

TYPE OF VARICOSE VEIN	GENERAL SYMPTOMS	WORSE FROM	BETTER FOR	REMEDY NAME
Tight, aching sensation in affected veins	- When more differentiating symptoms are missing, this is a good remedy for easing the aching pain of varicose veins - Circulation is sluggish with a tendency to develop chilblains	- Touch - Pressure - Jarring movement - During the day	- During the night	**Hamamelis**
Right-sided varicose veins that date from pregnancy	- Generally poor circulation with very cold hands and feet that are prone to develop chilblains - Sitting and/or standing may make pain and discomfort worse - Weepy and in need of sympathy and attention when in pain	- After becoming chilled and damp - Hot, stuffy rooms - Heavy covers on the bed - Rest	- Gentle exercise - Being in the fresh air - Cool compresses - Taking clothes off	**Pulsatilla**
Protruding purple veins that are more noticeable on the left leg	- Varicose veins may be more tender on the left side, or pains may move from the left to the right - Constricted, throbbing sensations are aggravated by wearing restrictive clothing or getting overheated	- Being immobile - On waking from sleep - Before a period - During the menopause	- Start of a period - Letting cool air get to the legs - Applying cool compresses to the painful areas	**Lachesis**
Serious aching in varicose veins with very restless legs	- Aching in veins is especially problematic when trying to rest in bed at night; legs move about constantly in an effort to find a comfortable position - Legs feel swollen, stiff and tired	- Sudden, jarring movements - Light touch - After marked physical effort	- Resting with the head lower than the body	**Arnica**
Burning, itching discomfort with varicose veins	- Varicose veins affect the groin and genitals, in addition to the legs - Burning sensations and associated cramping pains in calf muscles are especially troublesome at night	- Becoming overheated - Stuffy rooms - Moving	- Opening windows to let in cool, fresh air - Being fanned - After sound rest - Cool compresses	**Carbo veg**

homeopathy

139

cellulite or 'orange peel' skin

Every year, in all the glossy health and fashion magazines, pages and pages are written on how to master those bumpy bits of skin on the thighs, belly and upper arms. Indeed, if you are ever in doubt that cellulite is a very big business, just take a stroll through your local high street pharmacy and count the number of cellulite-busting gels, creams and body scrubs that are flying off the shelves. Interestingly, medical opinion is somewhat divided over the cellulite issue, as while many view it as an indication of significant toxic overload, others treat is as a troublesome cosmetic curse.

Although in some conventional medical circles there are still those who insist that there's no such thing as cellulite – it's just fat by another name – there are many complementary therapists who would disagree. They see the presence of significant patches of cellulite as an indicator that the body's lymphatic system is sluggish and in need of stimulation. As the lymphatic system forms a key component of the intricate network of organs that make up the immune system, the basic defence mechanism of the body against developing illness, it does make sense to find ways of supporting the efficient circulation of lymphatic fluid.

It is important to point out that being a slim, healthy build is no protection against developing cellulite on the buttocks and upper thighs. However, having a history of yo-yo dieting can play a part as the frequent and radical changes in weight loss and weight gain make it difficult for the skin to keep its elastic, smooth texture. Aside from constant dieting, any of the following are also thought to contribute to the presence of cellulite:

- **A chronically sedentary lifestyle that revolves around driving to work, sitting at a desk all day and collapsing in front of the television at night**
- **A diet that's high in alcohol, coffee, sugary drinks and convenience foods places a toxic load on the system as these are rich sources of unhealthy fats, refined sugar and preservatives**
- **A lack of a regular skin maintenance regime to ensure healthy skin tone and texture, e.g. exfoliation in, or before the shower**

As with so many of the skin conditions already discussed, any programme that's aiming to reduce the appearance of cellulite is going to focus on improving the body's general state of health. Measures of this kind will lighten the toxic burden on the body and improve energy levels, resulting in an overall sense of enhanced vitality as the body becomes less dependent on chemical stimulants to keep up the pace.

practical self-help

❧ Dry-skin body brushing on a daily basis gently and efficiently stimulates the flow of lymphatic fluid. Get into the habit of moving over the surface of the skin with a natural bristle brush for a few minutes before showering in the morning, and/or bathing in the evening. For best results find a long-handled, dry brush that allows you to reach otherwise hard-to-get-to areas and brush the skin with long, sweeping movements. Use firm, but not harsh pressure, moving up the fronts and backs of the legs and thighs, buttocks and belly, before moving up the arms and shoulders, not forgetting to concentrate on the upper arms but avoiding any areas of irritated or broken skin. Apart from encouraging efficient lymphatic fluid movement, this also has a gentle exfoliating effect on the skin, improving its appearance as well as encouraging body moisturisers to be absorbed more effectively.

❧ Taking regular, rhythmical exercise is very important as the contraction and relaxation of the muscles in the arms and legs keeps the flow of lymphatic fluid moving efficiently through the channels of the lymphatic system.

❧ Lymphatic drainage massage can both effectively prevent and manage cellulite by stimulating more efficient movement of lymphatic fluid.

❧ As with so many other skin conditions, diet and lifestyle are essential. Cut down drastically on cigarettes, alcohol, caffeinated drinks, high-fat, processed foods, red meat (especially highly processed varieties such as salami, bacon and sausages) and food and drinks that are full of white, refined sugar.

❧ Drink plenty of water on a daily basis to maintain healthy skin tone. Aim to have five large glasses a day and more in high summer temperatures when you lose more fluid to perspiration.

❧ Avoid soaking in very hot baths as they can aggravate problems with cellulite.

Generally speaking, there are no specific anti-cellulite remedies but seeking treatment from a homeopathic practitioner can be a helpful strategy if your ultimate aim is to get the body working in a more balanced, efficient way. If you have a marked tendency to cellulite, combined with a sluggish immune system, you will probably also suffer from a number of minor infections, such as colds and sore throats, throughout the year.

Therefore, in addition to appropriate homeopathic prescribing, most practitioners will be able to suggest positive lifestyle changes that will benefit your system as a whole. When this happens, cosmetic improvements such as healthier, smoother skin texture should become visible within a broader context of healthier energy levels, more balanced emotions and greater mental focus.

poor-quality, dry hair

As with the appearance of your skin, the quality and overall texture of your hair can say a great deal about your base-line level of health. Common problems that become visible when hair quality is falling short of its best can include any of the following:

- **Dry hair that splits or breaks easily**
- **Lack of gloss and shine**
- **Poor hair volume**
- **Falling hair that leads to an overall thin or patchy appearance**

Conventional medical support tends to concentrate on the more extreme kind of hair problems, like alopecia, which causes hair to fall out in circular patches anywhere over the crown or sides of the head. Any of the strategies suggested below will be most helpful in reversing a mild to moderate decline in hair quality. However, as elsewhere, more established or severe hair problems will have a better chance with a trained practitioner in complementary medicine. When choosing a therapist, try and locate one who also has a working knowledge of nutritional medicine. The connection between good nutrition and healthy hair is very strong and this should guarantee you the best of both worlds.

practical self-help

✎ Consult your hairdresser. If poor hair quality is the result of aggressive hair colouring, or overusing appliances, such as hairdryers and straighteners on too hot a setting, then action needs to be taken on this level first. If you are really attached to the colour of your hair dye, switch to a more natural product that contains fewer chemicals. Also, when drying your hair, first blot it gently with a towel, use a cooler setting on the hairdryer and avoid pulling or dragging the hair shaft when damp.

✎ If you are under a lot of stress, find the time in your daily routine to take up regular exercise or consult a counsellor who specialises in management strategies.

✎ Vitamin B complex and zinc have a beneficial effect on hair quality and texture so if you are feeling run down, take a good quality multimineral and multivitamin supplement while you get yourself back on track.

✎ Use gentle hair products that are compatible with the pH value of the hair. Ask your hairdresser's advice about the most suitable formula for your own hair type, avoiding any products that are likely to have a harsh or drastic detergent effect.

puffy eyes or dark circles under the eyes

Mild, infrequent episodes of swelling around the eyes, or dark circles underneath the eyes can be one of the most common signs of a night (or a few!) out on the tiles. Other common triggers of tired looking, puffy eyes can include any of the following:

- **An allergic reaction to pollen, house dust mite, make-up or cosmetics**
- **Crying**
- **Having too little, or not refreshing enough sleep for too long a period of time**
- **A few drinks too many**
- **Puffy eyes with itching, redness and sensitivity would suggest conjunctivitis**

practical self-help

☙ Puffy eyes can be an indication that the eliminatory organs, such as the kidneys, are under strain so drink plenty of water and avoid foods that are high in chemical flavourings, preservatives and food colourings as well as salt, sugar and refined carbohydrates.

☙ If puffy eyes are part of a general tendency to fluid retention, avoid foods that are high in salt. Drink dandelion tea or sprinkle liberal amounts of fresh parsley on your food as they both have a gentle fluid-balancing effect.

☙ Dark circles that have appeared due to sleep disturbance are best dealt with by attending to the underlying problem. See the relevant section on page 99.

☙ Periodic episodes of puffy eyes that are triggered by an allergy, such as hay fever, are best dealt with by consulting a homeopathic practitioner who can treat the underlying imbalance. This may involve two or three years of treatment in the autumn and winter months to prepare the body for the summer but it is almost guaranteed to reduce the misery of recurrent hay fever and to release you from your dependency on antihistamines.

☙ A quick pick-me-up for tired, puffy eyes: soak a couple of cotton wool pads in a cool solution of diluted Euphrasia tincture, wring them out and rest them on closed eyes for ten minutes while you put your feet up.

CAUTION!

If recurrent symptoms of puffy eyes are combined with puffy ankles, fingers, and a tendency to get very tired and breathless from only slight exertion, you should seek prompt medical advice

Homeopathic Support Table overleaf

TYPE OF PUFFY EYES	GENERAL SYMPTOMS	WORSE FROM	BETTER FOR	REMEDY NAME
Puffy eyes with marked sensitivity to warmth	- Skin around the eyes looks puffy and pinkish, as though fluid is trapped under the skin - Symptoms appear quickly and are most noticeable after sleep and rest	- Contact with warmth in any form - Lying down	- Cool compresses - Cool bathing of the puffy areas - Gentle exercise	**Apis**
Puffy, tired eyes that have been triggered by disturbed, pre-menstrual sleep	- Puffy eyes make an appearance at ovulation and get steadily worse until the onset of the period. Once this happens, puffiness goes down almost immediately - Sleep is very poor with a tendency to be anxious, restless, hot and sweaty at night	- After mid-cycle - Waking from sleep - Becoming overheated	- Coolness, in any form - The onset of a period	**Lachesis**
Puffy eyes with a marked craving for salty foods	- A tendency to puffiness around the eyes is combined with skin that is very dry in some patches and oily in others - Fluid imbalance is most noticeable before and after a period - A tendency to very sensitive skin is associated with a history of allergies	- Being in hot, sunny conditions for too long - Bright sunlight - Too many convenience foods and snacks that have a high salt content	- Cool bathing and cool compresses - Gentle exercise in the fresh air	**Natrum mur**
Puffy, tired eyes that follow a night of too much partying	- Eyes look red and baggy, or have dark circles as a result of too little sleep, too much junk food and alcohol and too many cigarettes - The whole system feels toxic and in need of a thorough cleansing	- Coffee - Feeling stressed and under pressure - First thing in the morning - Constipation	- Having a few hours of sound sleep - Relaxation - Achieving a satisfactory bowel movement	**Nux vomica**

homeopathy and winter conditions

This is the chapter to turn to if you know that every winter you and your family are prone to colds, coughs and/or sore throats in quick succession. Minor as these conditions are, it undoubtedly makes the prospect of the winter months extra depressing if you know you have one sniffle after another to look forward to.

The good news is that you can take plenty of proactive steps to give you the best chance of fighting off minor winter infections. And if you are unlucky enough to catch something even in spite of your best preventative efforts, this chapter also outlines the steps you can take to shorten the duration of the misery and reduce the risk of developing unpleasant complications like a tickly cough or bout of catarrh that just refuses to clear up. Best of all, you'll be able to face another winter feeling empowered rather than helpless and this in itself should get you through those gloomy, chilly months.

coughs

A nasty cough often follows a heavy cold or bout of flu and the congestion in the chest can trigger any combination of the following symptoms:

- **Tightness and/or muscle pain in the chest**
- **Coughing that is dry and irritating or very loose and mucusy**
- **Severe coughing spasms that can lead to gagging or actual vomiting**

The sort of coughs that will benefit from the following self-help are those that are acute, uncomplicated and not linked to a chronic chest problem such as asthma. Chest infections are always a danger for asthmatics and so with these cases it would be a good idea to see your doctor, ideally in combination with treatment from a complementary therapist.

practical self-help

❧ Avoid dairy foods where possible as they can make congestion worse – as a rule, don't eat any dairy if you are experiencing any kind of cold symptom in the chest, sinuses or ears.

❧ Lying flat at night encourages congestion to sit on the lungs so try sleeping propped up on two or three pillows, provided this feels comfortable for your neck.

❧ Steamy atmospheres are good for easing a dry, tickly cough, especially those that are noticeably worse for inhaling dry, cold air so make the time to have a long, hot shower or lean over a basin of steaming water.

❧ Garlic has a well-deserved reputation as a natural antibacterial and antiviral agent and can therefore assist the immune system in fighting infection. It is very difficult to consume enough raw garlic for it to have a therapeutic effect so take a good-quality supplement of concentrated garlic extract is much more practical. Taking a high-potency tablet once a day or a lower dose three times a day at mealtimes, as this should buffer any digestive repeating that can sometimes happen a few hours later.

❧ Massage a soothing essential oil blend into the chest and throat. Add four drops of tea tree, sweet green myrtle or eucalyptus (not to be used in massage blends for babies or toddlers) to two teaspoonfuls of carrier oil and massage around the chest and throat with warm hands, four times a day until the cough has cleared. (Be aware, however, that inhaling these essential oils may interfere with the medicinal action of a homeopathic remedy and so avoid using this blend too close to taking a dose.)

❧ Coughing is the body's way of removing irritating substances, excess secretions and foreign objects from air passages and is a healthy, protective mechanism as well as an important part of the healing process. It is therefore not a good idea to artificially suppress the cough reflex with medication as this can greatly hamper recovery.

CAUTION!

• If there's any suspicion that a coughing spasm is the result of inhaling a foreign body – common causes in children include pushing tiny objects up the nose that accidentally enter the windpipe – lose no time in seeking emergency medical help

IF THE FOLLOWING SYMPTOMS ARE MILD, CONSULT YOUR DOCTOR. HOWEVER, TAKE THE PATIENT TO THE NEAREST A&E DEPARTMENT IF THEY ARE CAUSING DISTRESS AND ESCALATING IN SEVERITY:

• Coughing that's accompanied by severe chest pain
• Marked wheezing or laboured breathing
• Drowsiness and/or confusion that date from the onset of a severe cough

TYPE OF COUGH	GENERAL SYMPTOMS	WORSE FROM	BETTER FOR	REMEDY NAME
Dry, irritating cough in the throat or upper chest	- Constant tickling in the throat triggers frustrating coughing spasms that lead to muscle pain in the chest - A constant desire to take a deep breath intensifies the coughing and leads to headaches	- The least movement - Overheated rooms - Taking a deep breath - Light touch	- Firm pressure to painful muscles - Sitting up - Keeping as still as possible - Resting	**Bryonia**
Coughing bouts set off by any light touch to the throat	- Raw, burning sensations in the chest intensify as a result of inhaling deeply - When phlegm is raised as a result of choking coughing spasms it looks frothy and clear - Exhausted from constantly interrupted sleep	- Taking a deep breath - Moving from one temperature to another - Eating - Inhaling cold air	- Wrapping up well - Covering the mouth	**Rumex**
Harsh-sounding cough with stringy mucus that is difficult to raise	- Cough develops in the established stage of a cold, accompanied by pain and congestion in the sinuses - Because of the muscular effort required to raise the mucus, pains radiate to the back and shoulders during a coughing spasm	- Cold, damp air - Waking from sleep - Alcohol - Bending over	- Warmth - Pressure to painful areas - Moving around	**Kali bich**
Established stage of a cough with yellow-coloured phlegm and painless loss of voice	- Tightness and pressure in the chest with an alternating loose and dry cough that is set off by moving from one temperature to another - Due to the effort of coughing stomach muscles feel strained	- Morning and evening - Lying on the left side - When speaking - Getting anxious - Strong smells	- Massage - Rest - Relaxing company - After a sound sleep	**Phosphorus**
Lingering cough with thick, greenish phlegm that comes from the chest and throat	- A dry, tickly night time cough becomes loose and productive as soon as you get up - The whole head feels full of mucus; phlegm tastes salty, buttery or unpleasantly sweet	- Stuffy, overheated rooms - At night - Resting - After eating	- Gentle movement in the open air - Fresh air - Sympathy and attention	**Pulsatilla**

homeopathy

●

earaches

Although earaches are generally more of a frequent occurrence in childhood, this painful condition can sometimes afflict adults as a complication of a heavy cold, especially if there was a tendency when young. Common symptoms can include any of the following:

- **Sharp or throbbing pain in the ears; limited to one side, or affecting both at once**
- **A general sense of feeling unwell, dizzy or feverishness**
- **Diminished hearing from fullness in the ear**
- **A thin, thick, coloured or bloody discharge that trickles out from the affected ear**
- **The first tell-tale sign of a developing ear problem in a baby or toddler is noticeable pulling or rubbing of the ears**

If an ear infection is confirmed by your doctor, you are likely to be given a prescription of antibiotics and possibly also ear drops. Any of the following measures can do a great deal to resolve a mild to moderate, one-off episode of earache, provided the situation is caught early enough – you ideally need to take action at the first twinge of pain or within two to three hours of its appearance. For more recurrent or severe problems, especially where babies and young children under the age of seven are involved, it would be beneficial to consult an experienced homeopathic practitioner and maybe also a cranial osteopath.

practical self-help

❧ Always make sure the ears are covered before going out in sharp, cold winds.

❧ Always avoid getting your ears wet when you have an ear infection or earache.

❧ Apply a warm compress to painful ears. Wrap a soft cloth or towel around a small hot water bottle, or wring out a hot, clean flannel and hold against the affected side.

❧ If your ear feels full and waxy as well as sore, never have a poke about with a foreign body such as a cotton bud as this can inadvertently cause damage. Instead, put a drop or two of almond oil in the ear on five consecutive nights and then go to your doctor surgery to have the ear examined and possibly syringed to clean out excess wax.

CAUTION!

IF ANY OF THE FOLLOWING OCCUR, CONSULT YOUR DOCTOR:

- **If drowsiness, stiffness of the neck or a general sense of malaise are also pronounced**
- **If ear pain is combined with any sign of dehydration in babies; tell-tale symptoms include drowsiness, reduced urine output, sunken eyes and/or very dry skin texture**
- **If there are signs of a pus formation or a discharge trickling out of the ear**

TYPE OF EARACHE	GENERAL SYMPTOMS	WORSE FROM	BETTER FOR	REMEDY NAME
Ear pain that develops quickly after exposure to sharp, cold winds	- Wakes in the night following exposure to cold winds feeling generally feverish and restless with ear pain - The body may feel cool while the head feels hot and feverish - Panicky and intolerant of pain	- Lying on painful side - Loud noise - Being disturbed from sleep - Extreme variation of temperature	- Breaking into a sweat - Comfortable warmth	**Aconite**
Fast-developing ear pain with localised heat and tenderness	- A rapidly-developing sense of feverishness - Symptoms may be limited to the right side, or feel worse on this side - Irritable and bad-tempered with pain	- Being disturbed - Becoming chilled - Jarring - Exposure to bright light	- Resting propped up in bed - Warm compresses	**Belladonna**
Rapid onset of ear pain that's less severe than symptoms needing Belladonna	- Drawing, itching pains in the ear that are either more severe on, or are limited to, the left side - Complexion may look unusually pale or flushed	- Cool air - Touch to painful area - During the night - Exposure to loud noise	- Cool compresses locally applied - Resting	**Ferrum phos**
Ear pain that's combined with a sore throat and swollen glands	- Pain develops during the established stage of a cold, which produces lots of thick, yellowish mucus - Sensitivity to cold is extreme, especially to cold air	- Becoming chilled - Lying on the painful side - During the night	- Keeping as warmly wrapped up as possible - Resting	**Hepar sulph**
Ear problems that come on after getting wet	- A sense of fullness and discomfort in the ear can be the result of mucus congestion left behind by a heavy cold - A marked intolerance to getting overheated - Weepy and emotional when in discomfort	- Resting - During the night - Humid conditions - Lack of contact with fresh air	- Cool drinks - Walking outside - Cool compresses - After a good cry	**Pulsatilla**

homeopathy

sinus problems

Although everyone has two sets of sinuses, located above the eyes and around the area of the cheekbones, most of the time they thankfully don't make their presence felt in the form of pain or congestion. However, for people who are prone to recurrent head colds in the winter, when the micro-organisms responsible for the cold spread and infect the mucus membranes in the narrow sinus cavities, it causes swelling, which traps the infected mucus and leads to a build up of painful pressure. Symptoms of inflamed sinuses (sinusitis) are debilitating and unpleasant and can include any of the following:

- **Severe headaches that lodge above the eyes, affecting both sides equally, or just one**
- **Throbbing pains in the cheekbones or bridge of the nose that are especially severe when bending forward**
- **Congestion in the nose, or a sense of the nose being uncomfortably blocked**
- **Pain in the sinuses on blowing the nose**
- **Thick, yellow or green mucus that can taste and smell unpleasant**
- **Pain in the upper jaw caused by jarring movement. This can be mistaken for toothache**

Conventional treatment relies on giving courses of antibiotics to relieve symptoms of infection. If bouts of sinusitis are becoming frequent and/or severe, a minor surgical procedure may also be required to encourage the sinuses to drain more effectively. While the following measures can help to speed up recovery from a one-off, acute episode of sinus inflammation, recurrent problems would benefit greatly from professional complementary treatment.

practical self-help

❧ Avoid dairy products and sugary foods as they aggravate congestion.

❧ Resist the urge to give your nose an almighty blow in the hope that it will clear blocked sinuses, as this can make the pain and discomfort much worse.

❧ Use a humidifier in dry, central-heated environments.

❧ Take a supplement of concentrated garlic extract. Follow the dosage advice on the packet and always take with food in order to buffer any digestive repeating.

❧ For the duration of the infection, take a combined vitamin C and zinc formula supplement that provides both nutrients in a measured dose. If you feel another episode coming on, resume taking this supplement at the first twinge of discomfort.

❧ Make a decongestant blend from two drops of pine, eucalyptus and sweet marjoram added to two teaspoons of carrier oil and massage gently around the nostrils and the throat. (N.B. This blend is not suitable for babies or toddlers and, for adults, it is unwise to use it too close to taking a remedy, in case it interferes with the medicinal action.)

TYPE OF SINUS PROBLEM	GENERAL SYMPTOMS	WORSE FROM	BETTER FOR	REMEDY NAME
One-sided sinus pain with tired, tender feeling around and behind the eyes	- Strong sense of nasal congestion and obstruction especially in the evening and at night - When mucus does appear, it's yellow-coloured and possibly blood-streaked - Nasal passages feel swollen and are hypersensitive to smells	- Lying on the tender side - Lying flat on the back - On getting up - Evenings	- Sound rest - Massage - Splashing the face with cool water	**Phosphorus**
Sinusitis with pain that lodges at the bridge of the nose	- Nasal mucus is very difficult to expel because of its stringy, ropy texture - Mucus discharges are also likely to be green in colour, leading to a persistent nasty smell in the nose for the duration of infection	- Breathing in cold, damp air - Sleep - Bending forward - Alcohol	- Warmth in any form (locally applied or general atmosphere) - Firm pressure to sensitive area - Motion	**Kali bich**
Painful sinuses that react very badly to inhaling cold air	- Sneezing and an irritating sense of obstruction in the nose are triggered, or made noticeably worse, for contact with cold air. - Nasal mucus is characteristically thick and yellowish-green in colour - Touchy and short-fused	- During the night - Making any sort of physical effort - Touch - Being disturbed	- Warm, moist air	**Hepar sulph**
Sinus headaches that are set off or made more intense by stuffy, airless rooms	- Sinus problems characteristically follow a lingering cold with residual cough and swollen glands - Nasal obstruction is worst at night, while the nose starts running when up and about in the morning - Weepy and in need of sympathy when in pain	- During the night - Rest - Contact with warmth - Feeling neglected	- Taking a gentle walk in the fresh air - Cool compresses applied to the tender areas - After a good cry	**Pulsatilla**

homeopathy

●

sore throats and tonsillitis

The nature of a sore throat can vary quite dramatically, with some involving nothing more than localised pain and discomfort for a day or two at the beginning of a cold, while others taking the form of full-blown tonsillitis. The latter is a particularly unpleasant illness that affects the whole system and gives rise to any of the following symptoms.

- **High temperature**
- **Severe swelling and pain in the throat**
- **Vomiting**
- **Painful, swollen glands in the neck**
- **Headache**
- **Weariness and exhaustion**

practical self-help

❧ Increase your daily intake of vitamin C-rich foods and drinks in order to provide extra support for the immune system in fighting infection. Berries, citrus fruit, green, leafy vegetables, peppers, tomatoes, and lots of salad are all good sources, but if this doesn't appeal, take a course of slow-release vitamin C supplement (500mgs) every morning and evening until the infection has cleared up.

❧ Rest as much as possible in a smoke-free environment at a stable temperature.

❧ Drink lots of fluids, especially if you have a fever. Avoid diuretic beverages such as tea and coffee and instead drink generous amounts of filtered or still mineral water, herbal teas, fresh fruit juices and hot lemon and honey toddies.

❧ Sucking glycerine pastilles can give temporary relief to a sore throat and calm an irritating cough that is often triggered by a feeling of dryness. However, if you are taking homeopathic medicines, avoid lozenges or pastilles that contain strong aromatic flavours. Homeopathic remedies begin to work as they are absorbed by the mucus membranes in the mouth (in other words, you don't have to wait for them to be broken down by the stomach) and therefore strong flavours can potentially antidote their effectiveness.

❧ Gargle with a dilution of Calendula and Hypericum tincture (one part tincture to ten parts boiled cooled water) or, alternatively, use a combination of sage, cider vinegar and honey. Add one teaspoonful of sage to a medium-sized cup of warm water, leave to stand for a minute before straining and then add one teaspoonful of cider vinegar and honey.

❧ Gently rub a soothing massage into the tender area of the throat. Add three drops of eucalyptus and three drops of tea tree essential oils to two teaspoonfuls of carrier oil. However, for full-blown tonsillitis, seek the advice of an aromatherapist because of the potential severity of the symptoms.

TYPE OF SORE THROAT	GENERAL SYMPTOMS	WORSE FROM	BETTER FOR	REMEDY NAME
Fast developing sore throat with feverishness and dry, flushed skin	- Painful swollen throat and glands are worse or only affect the right side - Craves citrus-flavoured drinks but swallowing is painful - Bright red appearance to the throat - Cranky when feeling ill	- Becoming chilled - When speaking - Swallowing - Jarring motion	- Rest - Lying propped up in bed	**Belladonna**
Sore throats and swollen glands are especially painful on waking	- Pain and swelling in throat and glands may be limited to, or be more severe on, the left side - Throat feels tight, swollen and constricted - Swallowing food is curiously easier that 'empty' swallowing	- Warm drinks - The slightest touch or pressure on the throat (e.g. from a poloneck jumper or scarf)	- Cold drinks - Loosening clothes around the neck - Eating - As the day goes on	**Lachesis**
Sore throat with sharp, fish-bone type sensation that may be more intense on the right side	- Established stage of cold or slow-developing sore throat with swollen glands - Signs of ulceration on the throat and accompanying congestion in the nose, sinuses and/or chest that looks a yellowy-green colour	- Cold draughts - Undressing - Making any physical effort - Being touched - At night	- Contact with moist, steamy air - Keeping warm	**Hepar sulph**
Established stage of sore throat with severe swelling of the glands in the neck	- Throbbing pains and discomfort of the throat and glands is more pronounced on the right side - Localised burning pain is made worse from drinking hot liquids and swallowing - Throat looks bluish-red with possible dotting with greyish-white spots on tonsils	- Humidity - Making any physical effort - Contact with warmth - Sipping warm drinks	- Taking it very easy	**Phytolacca**

homeopathy

●

1 5 3

CAUTION!

Seek medical advice if a lingering and severe sore throat is combined with feverishness, and noticeable pain and swelling of the glands in the neck, and/or the armpits and groin

flu

Going through a full-blown bout of flu is a really nasty business that will make you feel very ill for anything up to two weeks. You can certainly expect a genuine flu bug to confine you to bed for several days, when you are likely to experience any combination of the following symptoms:

- **Feverishness and sweating**
- **Generalised aching with severe headache**
- **Chills that run up and down the body with shivering**
- **Coughing spasms**
- **Swollen, painful glands and sore throat**
- **Congestion in the nose, throat, ears and chest**
- **Lack of appetite with possible nausea**
- **Complete exhaustion**

Conventional medical advice consists of taking it as easy as possible, keeping fluid intake up, taking painkillers to soothe pain and regulate body temperature and maybe also cough medicines and decongestants, depending on the symptoms that are causing distress.

The following advice can be invaluable in supporting you through a bout of flu and giving you the best chance of a speedy recovery with the minimum risk of complications.

practical self-help

❧ In the early, feverish stage, the priority is to drink lots of fluids, rather than forcing food down when you don't feel hungry. Instead of 'keeping your strength up', this can have the counterproductive effect of raising your temperature further.

❧ Keep the ambient temperature as stable as possible.

❧ At the first sign of illness, such as a general sense of exhaustion or shivering, or something more specific, like a sore throat, act promptly and take a vitamin C supplement. A suitable dose would be 500mgs of slow-release vitamin C, taken morning and evening for the duration of infection.

❧ Once you start eating again, increase your vitamin C quota by including foods that provide naturally healthy sources of this immune-system-boosting nutrient.

❧ If you know that past episodes of flu have left you battling with a sinus or chest infection, take a garlic supplement at the earliest stage of infection.

❧ Because the liver is one of the body's major detox organs, it makes sense to strain the liver as little as possible when you have an infection. Avoid convenience foods that contain hefty amounts of chemical additives and preservatives and alcohol in any form.

❧ Rest up in bed and sleep if this is what your body is telling you to do.

TYPE OF FLU	GENERAL SYMPTOMS	WORSE FROM	BETTER FOR	REMEDY NAME
Classic slow-developing flu symptoms with marked exhaustion	- Feels off colour for several days with gradual emergence of aching muscles and chills that run up and down the spine - Eyes look droopy and heavy with headache and dizziness - Irritable and depressed when ill	- Any physical effort - Becoming chilled - Getting too hot	- Breaking into a sweat - Contact with fresh air - Passing water helps relieve the headache	**Gelsemium**
Severe flu symptoms with deep aching in the bones	- Muscles feel bruised with terrible aching in the long bones of the legs and the arms - Constant coughing causes muscle soreness in the chest, with general restlessness, weakness and queasiness	- Lying on aching muscles - In the morning - Feeling chilled - The thought, sight or smell of food	- Breaking into a sweat - Relief of vomiting - Distraction	**Eupatorium perfoliatum**
Flu with severe sore throat that makes it difficult to swallow solid food	- Sore, aching muscles - Sense of heaviness and weakness in the body but with alert mind - Restless, but so weak that any movement makes exhaustion worse	- Moist heat - After waking - Becoming chilled - Becoming too hot		**Baptisia**
Established phase of flu with swollen glands and severe sore throat	- Pain in the throat and glands with a noticeable increase in the amount of saliva in the mouth - Mucus is thick, yellowish-green in colour and tastes unpleasant - Anxiety and restlessness are worse during the night	- Breaking into a sweat - Exposure to damp - Getting too hot or too chilled	- Moderate comfortable temperature - Resting	**Mercurius**
Last stages of flu with congestion in the nose, sinuses, ears and/or chest	- Restless and uncomfortable when resting in bed with a real desire to get out in the fresh air - Mucus is thick, green and causes a lot of queasiness - The mouth is dry but without thirst - Generally chilly but becoming hot causes distress	- Stuffy rooms - Rest - In the evening - During the night - Feeling neglected	- Fresh air - Well-ventilated rooms - Sips of cool drinks - After a good cry	**Pulsatilla**

catarrh

This irritating condition doesn't necessarily limit itself to the autumn and winter months but it can be noticeably worse at these times of the year. Common symptoms can include any of the following:

- **A blocked or runny nose, or constant alternation between the two**
- **Coughing**
- **Blocked or painful ears**
- **A persistent tendency to have to hawk or clear the throat at regular intervals**

The conventional medical solution concentrates on decongestant drugs in the hope that the condition will disperse. Any of the following measures can be very helpful in relieving the odd, mild bout of catarrh, and can all be used safely in combination with any conventional treatment that may be necessary. As always, more established, severe or chronic tendencies to catarrh should be referred to a homeopathic practitioner in order to address the underlying constitutional imbalance.

practical self-help

❧ Avoid catarrh-aggravating foods such as dairy products or anything that contains a high proportion of refined, white sugar.

❧ Take regular exercise in the fresh air to clear the nasal passages.

❧ Avoid contact with cigarette smoke wherever, and whenever, possible as this only irritates the mucus membranes of the nose and throat.

❧ Eat plenty of antioxidant-rich food, such as red, yellow, dark green and orange fruit and vegetables together with generous helpings of fresh garlic and drink plenty of filtered or still mineral water.

❧ Make a decongestant aromatherapy blend that can be used as a gentle back and chest rub in the morning and evening. Add four drops of eucalyptus and lavender essential oils to two teaspoons of carrier oil. For a simpler version to unblock a congested nose, add few drops of either of these oils to a tissue and inhale gently. However, do not use this too close to taking a remedy as inhaling essential oils can sometimes interfere with the medicinal action of a homeopathic dose.

TYPE OF CATARRH	GENERAL SYMPTOMS	WORSE FROM	BETTER FOR	REMEDY NAME
Nasal catarrh that alternates between being thick and jelly-like and running like a tap	- Nose feels dry and blocked with occasional sneezing followed by a streaming nose with clear, watery discharge - Dry lips and cold sores	- Exposure to bright sunlight - Heat - During the summer (for instance in the hayfever season)	- Fresh, open air - Cool bathing or cool compresses - Rest - Rubbing	**Natrum mur**
Catarrh with sticky yellow discharge from the nose and throat	- Mucus discharges cause burning sensations in the affected areas - Lots of abortive sneezing with tingling in the nose - Upper lip feels sore as a result of a dripping nose	- Dry, cold weather - Windy weather - Humidity - Smoking	- Fresh air	**Arsenicum iod**
Ropy, stringy catarrh with pressure at bridge of the nose	- Catarrh looks thick and greenish yellow - Air from nostrils feels hot with nasty smell in the nose - Blocked nose with dry sensation and loss of sense of smell	- Cold, damp weather - In spring - Contact with fresh air - Stooping	- Warmth - Moving - Pressure locally applied	**Kali bich**
Thick yellow-green catarrh with dry mouth and coated tongue	- Catarrh sets in after a lingering head cold - Mucus discharges are thick, bland and unpleasant-tasting - Head feels as though it's filled with mucus when in a stuffy, overheated room	- In the evening and at night - Lying down - Fatty, dairy foods - Keeping still	- Walking in the fresh air - Cool compresses - Having a good cry - Sympathy and attention	**Pulsatilla**

homeopathy

●

157

colds

Although considered to be a very minor health problem, there's absolutely no doubt that the symptoms of a nasty cold can really put the dampener on your spirits and make it incredibly difficult to get on with the simplest daily tasks. Although the severity of symptoms will vary from one cold to another, in the early stages of a cold you are likely to sneeze a lot, feel generally out of sorts and have a dry, tickly sore throat and painful ears. In the more established stage of a cold, the following symptoms are common:

- **Swollen glands**
- **A dry and tickly or loose and productive cough**
- **Pain across the cheekbones and/or above the eyes**
- **Headaches**
- **Nasal congestion with mucus that may be thick and yellowish-green in colour**
- **Muffled hearing with a feeling of blocked-up ears**

practical self-help

❧ One of the most effective ways of fighting a cold in its early stages is to take it very easy so that all the energy that is needed to fight an acute infection isn't diverted elsewhere. However, if staying in bed just isn't an option, at least make sure that your environment is kept at a stable temperature as this also conserves the body's energy and avoids aggravating the symptoms.

❧ Taking Echinacea at the first sign of a sniffle can do an enormous amount to support the immune system and speed up recovery. Take according to the directions on the packaging for the duration of the cold or, for a good preventative measure, take for a day or two if you have any close contact with people who seem to be in the infectious stages of a cold.

❧ If your nostrils have become sore from frequently wiping a running nose, apply a little Calendula cream to soothe the skin.

❧ If congestion is a problem in the head and chest, cut down on dairy products and very sweet foods as they encourage the production of mucus and will therefore make the symptoms worse.

❧ Taking a vitamin C supplement may not prevent you catching a cold but it should at least shorten the duration of the infection. Choose a slow-release formula or take 500mgs morning and evening, as standard formulas are often excreted within a few hours of taking the supplement.

❧ Drinking plenty of water guards against low-grade dehydration which can make sore throats and headaches worse.

TYPE OF COLD	GENERAL SYMPTOMS	WORSE FROM	BETTER FOR	REMEDY NAME
Early stage of a cold that comes on after exposure to dry, cold winds	- Symptoms often come on after sleep with a sore throat, sensitive eyes and a dry or runny nose with clear, watery mucus - Restless with an overall intolerance of pain	- Touch or pressure - While sweating - During the night - Smoking	- Rest	**Aconite**
Initial stage of a cold with a rapidly developing high temperature	- Skin looks red and flushed with feverishness and feels very hot and dry - When this remedy is well indicated, symptoms come on abruptly and include a severe sore throat, swollen glands and ear pain	- Noise - Cold draughts - Bright light - Motion - Touch	- Being lightly covered - Resting - Being propped up in bed	**Belladonna**
Initial stage of a cold with earache and a sore throat	- Throat feels swollen and tender and swallowing is especially painful - Earache may cause slightly reduced hearing - Face looks alternately flushed and pale	- Jarring movement - Cold drinks - At night - Becoming chilled	- Cool compresses - Lying down	**Ferrum phos**
Head cold with thick yellow mucus	- Sore throat, swollen glands and possible sinus congestion - Sharp, sticking pains in the throat	- Cold draughts - Undressing - Touch or pressure - During the night - Physical effort	- Moist air - Wrapping up warmly	**Hepar sulph**

homeopathy

159

Homeopathic Support Table continued overleaf

TYPE OF COLD	GENERAL SYMPTOMS	WORSE FROM	BETTER FOR	REMEDY NAME
Head cold with nasal discharge that runs like a tap and then gets blocked	- When blocked, there is a feeling of dryness and obstruction high up in the nose - Lips become dry and cracked and cold sores are common - Bouts of sneezing are more severe for being in bright sunlight	- Attention and sympathy - Heat - Making an effort - Touch	- Fresh air - Contact with cool water - Cool compresses - Privacy	**Natrum mur**
Colds with scanty, clear nasal discharge that burns the nostrils	- Generally very chilly with burning pains in the throat and nose - Tightness in the chest with a dry, tickly cough that is eased by being propped up at night	- Lying flat - Making any physical effort - Becoming chilled - When alone	- Sips of warm drinks - Warm bathing - Company	**Arsenicum album**
Last stages of a cold with lots of thick, greenish-yellow mucus	- Chilly but feels uncomfortable and congested in warm, stuffy rooms - Mucus congestion makes the sinuses painful, while glands are sensitive and the ears muffled - Coughing bouts alternate between dry and tickly and loose and productive	- Overheated rooms - Dairy foods - Feeling neglected - At night - Rest	- Contact with fresh air - Gentle exercise of doors - After a good cry - Sympathy and attention	**Pulsatilla**

CAUTION!

IF ANY OF THE FOLLOWING OCCUR, CONSULT YOUR DOCTOR:

- **Marked feverishness (40°C/104°F) that develops in babies, toddlers or the elderly, especially if it is resistant to self-help measures**
- **Laboured or wheezing breathing**
- **Throat infections in anyone who has previously suffered from rheumatic fever**

homeopathy on holiday

Taking a homeopathic first-aid kit on holiday with you is one of the most practical things you can do to ensure that minor health problems don't interfere with an otherwise relaxing break. The whole family can benefit from effective homeopathic prescribing and the following tried-and-tested remedies will particularly be a godsend for anyone travelling with babies, toddlers or young children.

food poisoning

Food poisoning is really the last thing you want when you are on holiday and yet, unfortunately, it can hit at any time and often in surprising locations. After travelling in Morocco, Spain, France, Italy, Australia and New Zealand with absolutely no digestive worries, I was regrettably struck down by a particularly unpleasant bout of food poisoning in Devon! Triggers can vary but often include ice in drinks made from contaminated water, salad or fruit washed in suspect water, infected meat or fish or perishable food that has been poorly stored and/or cooked. Common symptoms include any of the following:

- **Vomiting**
- **Stomach pains and discomfort**
- **Diarrhoea**
- **Abdominal pain and discomfort**
- **Extreme listlessness and exhaustion**

practical self-help

✎ The first priority, especially if vomiting and diarrhoea occur together, is to keep fluid intake up and this is particularly important for babies, young children and the elderly.
✎ Don't force food on anyone in the twenty-four to forty-eight hours following a bout of food poisoning as overloading the digestive tract when it's not ready can cause more harm than good; drink fluids instead.

❧ In the early stages of food poisoning, avoid giving any medication that is designed to stop the vomiting and diarrhoea reflexes as it is these that need to rid the body of any undesirable bugs as quickly and effectively as possible. Anti-diarrhoea drugs, for example, will only make it harder for the body to deal with the problem efficiently.

❧ Once recovery is well under way, choose foods that are soothing to the digestive tract, such as soups, rice, fish, lightly cooked vegetables, salads, and soothing herb teas. However, avoid anything with a high fat content, such as cheese, red meat and cream, all pulses like beans and lentils, alcohol, coffee and citrus fruit juices.

TYPE OF FOOD POISONING	GENERAL SYMPTOMS	WORSE FROM	BETTER FOR	REMEDY NAME
Severe, extremely watery diarrhoea that feels painless	- An explosive bout of diarrhoea is heralded by loud gurgling in the belly and results in weakness and nausea - Diarrhoea may be caused by eating too much fruit	- After eating - Moving about - Early in the morning - Before, during or after an episode of diarrhoea	- Massage - Lying on the belly	**Podophyllum**
Diarrhoea with severe discomfort from trapped wind	- Near to state of collapse with severe cramping pains and diarrhoea - Feels exhausted, clammy and chilly but craves contact with fresh, cool air - Intolerant of tight clothing, especially around the waist	- Becoming chilled - Stuffy, overheated rooms - Clothes that fit too snuggly	- Being fanned - Releasing wind - Resting with the feet slightly higher than the body	**Carbo veg**
Gushing, urgent bouts of diarrhoea that come on as soon as you wake up	- On first getting up, has to rush to the bathroom in order to pass violent, frothy diarrhoea - Bowel movements leave the anus feeling sore, inflamed and itchy - Because of the degree of discomfort there's a tendency to put off going until the very last moment	- Warm bathing - Getting hot in bed - Becoming chilled - Making any effort - Sugar	- Contact with fresh, cool air - Sweating - Moderate, regulated temperature	**Sulphur**

TYPE OF FOOD POISONING	GENERAL SYMPTOMS	WORSE FROM	BETTER FOR	REMEDY NAME
Food poisoning with vomiting and diarrhoea that occur together	- Exhausted but restless with vomiting and diarrhoea - Pale, anxious and sweaty - Small sips of a warm drink ease burning sensation in the stomach	- Cold, in any form - During the night - Alcohol	- Warmth, in any form - Rest - After breaking into a sweat	**Arsenicum album**
Vomiting and diarrhoea that occur together	- Exhausted, sweaty and prostrated with severity of symptoms - Unquenchable thirst for long, cold drinks that are forcibly vomited back up again - Icy cold sweats are especially drenching after vomiting or a bout of diarrhoea	- Taking fluids - Warmth - When passing a bowel movement - Sweating - At night	- Rest - Lying down - Contact with cool	**Veratrum album**
Burning pains in the stomach with desire for cold drinks	- Nausea and vomiting with craving for ice-cold drinks that are thrown up as soon as they get warmed in the stomach - Diarrhoea feels corrosive and burning as it's passed	- Warm drinks - Talking - Making any effort - Lying flat on the back	- Unbroken rest - Bathing the face in cold water	**Phosphorus**
Bad nausea that is not relieved by vomiting	- Continuous nausea that is aggravated by even the slightest movement - Bloated belly with spasmodic colicky pains - No thirst with frothy or mucus-streaked vomit	- Moving - Warmth - Vomiting	- Rest - Cold drinks - Closing the eyes - Contact with fresh air	**Ipecac**

homeopathy

163

CAUTION!

IF ANY OF THE FOLLOWING OCCUR, GET SWIFT MEDICAL ASSISTANCE:

- Drowsiness, dry skin, reduced urine output and/or sunken eyes
- Severe pain in the stomach or abdomen that doesn't improve within 24 hours
- Vomiting and/or diarrhoea that refuses to clear up within 48 hours

jet lag

Jet lag is caused by the body's inability to adjust rapidly to a new time zone and its severity is often influenced by the direction of travel, as the body seems to tolerate westward flights far better than eastward ones. The problems caused by jet lag can be unpleasant enough to upset the first day or two of a long awaited holiday, and make the coming back even more depressing than usual. The degree to which we suffer these symptoms is often determined by our constitutional susceptibility but any of the following are common features of the experience:

- **Sleep disturbance**
- **Exhaustion and sleepiness during the day**
- **Problems in mentally focusing and concentrating**
- **Suppressed appetite**
- **Constipation**

practical self-help

❧ Jet lag appears to be related to the escalating production of free radicals in the body and therefore it is a good idea to combat their destructive effect by increasing your intake of antioxidant nutrients. These include the vitamins A,C and E that are found in all bright red, yellow, orange and dark green fresh fruit and vegetables so eat at least five portions of these the day before and after a journey. Airline food isn't generally the healthiest so pack five servings of fruit in your hand luggage to eat during the trip.

❧ Make sure you keep fluid intake up as it is very easy to become dehydrated in the pressurised environment of an aeroplane and this can exaggerate symptoms of jet lag. However tempting the drinks trolley might look, it's definitely worth resisting alcohol, as it will only aggravate dehydration and contribute to sleep disturbance once you reach your destination.

❧ If you suffer from swollen feet and ankles on a long-haul flight, walk up and down the aisle every hour or so in order to keep your circulation moving and avoid heavily salted snacks such as crisps and nuts, which encourage the body to retain fluid.

❧ If you get to your destination during the day, resist the urge to have a nap on your arrival as this will give you a better chance of drifting off when you need to at night.

TYPE OF JET LAG	GENERAL SYMPTOMS	WORSE FROM	BETTER FOR	REMEDY NAME
Jet lag with inability to switch off and get to sleep	- Constant starting awake when drifting off to sleep - Feels exhausted and sluggish when it's time to get up - Total lack of appetite with nausea and constipation	- Coffee - Between midnight and 2a.m. - Smoking	- Peace and quiet - Resting	**Cocculus**
Jet lag with a feeling of being hungover	- Irritability, nausea, tension headaches and constipation - Aggravated by drinking alcohol and eating junk food on the flight	- Lack of sleep - Alcohol - Feeling constipated	- Peace and quiet - Rest - Passing a stool	**Nux vomica**

homeopathy

165

overindulgence

Everyone is understandably more relaxed about eating and drinking when away from the routine of home and therefore it's good to know that there's homeopathic support at hand for the times when overindulgence gets the better of you. A common mistake, however, is simply not to keep fluid intake up, especially when drinking alcohol, and so bear in mind that this could save you from a whole range of hangover-type evils.

Common symptoms of overindulgence can include any of the following, in varying degrees of severity:

- **Headache**
- **Nausea**
- **Indigestion**
- **Flatulence**
- **Loss of appetite**
- **Constipation or slight diarrhoea**
- **Fatigue and listlessness**
- **Irritability**

practical self-help

❧ The first steps to recovery include rehydrating the body and avoiding any indigestible foods that are too spicy, fatty or generally very rich. Drink still water at room temperature as the heavily iced varieties can make the stomach feel quite uncomfortable. For variety's sake, you can also have non-acidic fruit juice, such as apple, but avoid orange and grapefruit juice as their acidity can irritate an already sensitive stomach.

❧ If you are suffering from a bad hangover, stay away from alcohol for at least forty-eight hours in order for the liver to recover.

❧ Temporary queasiness can be eased by sipping a warm cup of ginger tea, or nibbling on a piece of crystallised ginger.

❧ If the headache is the major problem, rest in a quiet, cool room with your eyes shut and with a cool flannel covering the forehead. Applying a few drops of peppermint essential oil around the hairline can also feel soothing and reviving.

TYPE OF OVERINDULGENCE	GENERAL SYMPTOMS	WORSE FROM	BETTER FOR	REMEDY NAME
Classic overindulgence from too much, or an unwise mixture of alcohol	- Severe queasiness and headache that lodges at the back of the head and feels especially bad on waking the following morning - Feels like being sick would help but it takes a lot of retching to bring anything up - Irritable and short-fused	- Waking - Smoking too much - Too many coffees - Lack of rest - Unwise mixture of foods	- Rest - Sound sleep - Being sick - Passing a stool	**Nux vomica**
Overindulging on rich, fatty foods	- Nausea and headaches - Indigestion is especially uncomfortable overnight, when lying down or for jarring movement, like walking quickly on a hard surface	- In the evening and at night - Resting - Warm food and drink	- Sipping a cold drink - Small portions of light, cold foods, like salads - Contact with cool, fresh air - Taking a gentle stroll	**Pulsatilla**
Overindulging on high-fibre foods	- Acid indigestion and heartburn as a result of eating a large amount of fibre-rich foods - Lots of stomach bloating with noticeable rumbling, gurgling and production of wind	- Reaction to stress and tension - Tight clothes around the waist - Eating too quickly	- Loosening clothes - Passing wind - Sips of a warm drink and small amounts of hot food	**Lycopodium**

homeopathy

●

167

hives and allergic skin rashes

Anyone with sensitive skin needs to take particular care on holiday as being exposed to a hot sun is often enough to trigger a reaction. Take care that you use a suncream that will not aggravate the condition and consult a pharmacist before making your choice.

Common symptoms of a localised skin reaction can include any combination of the following:

- **Red, raised patches on the skin**
- **Severe itching**
- **Itchy areas look large and blotchy, or consist of a small, intensely itchy pinprick rash**
- **Affected areas are restricted to one area of the body, or move from one part to another over the course of a few days**
- **Cold sores on the face as a reaction to over-exposure to sunlight**

practical self-help

❧ The first priority should be to cool the skin down and protect the affected areas from further exposure to heat and sunlight. Keep them lightly covered with clothing made from linen, natural cotton or silk, which allows the skin to breathe and stay cool.

❧ If skin is itchy and stinging, bathe it first in a diluted Urtica urens tincture before applying Urtica urens cream. Dilute one part tincture in ten parts water (boiled, then cooled) and apply with a cotton wool pad. Pat dry before gently applying the cream. If your skin is especially reactive do a patch test: rub a small amount into the fine skin on the inside of the wrist, two or three times at hourly intervals and, if the skin takes it well, you can then use it more liberally.

CAUTION!

IF ANY OF THE FOLLOWING OCCUR, GET SWIFT MEDICAL ASSISTANCE:

- **Intense itching of the skin combined with breathing difficulties**
- **Problems with swallowing**
- **Any sign of rapid-developing swelling around the face, lips or throat**

TYPE OF SKIN REACTION	GENERAL SYMPTOMS	WORSE FROM	BETTER FOR	REMEDY NAME
Small, blistery, intensely itchy spots	- Maddeningly itchy spots cause particular distress at night, with restlessness and interrupted sleep - Skin reaction develops after getting chilled and wet with sensitivity of the skin to draughts of cool air	- Taking clothes off - Rest in bed - Making any physical effort	- Warm bathing - Very gentle movement - Stretching - Rubbing	**Rhus tox**
Large, pink blotches that emerge rapidly in response to heat	- Affected areas look pale, rosy pink and/or fluid-filled - Itchiness, combined with a stinging sensation, becomes much more distressing from contact with heat in any form	- Warmth - Rest - Being touched - Pressure	- Cool compresses - Taking clothes off - Exposure to cool air - Gentle movement in the fresh air	**Apis**
Small, itchy spots with burning sensation that's eased by warmth	- Very irritated spots that itch and burn violently, especially at night, which leads to great anxiety and restlessness in bed - Warmth in any form temporarily eases the distress	- Becoming cold or chilled - During the night - Lying on the affected areas - Making any physical effort	- Sitting propped up in bed - Being distracted - Warmth	**Arsenicum album**

homeopathy

●

leisure sickness

This is the smart new term that is used to describe the health problems that have a nasty habit of striking just at the moment when you begin to relax and unwind. Classic examples include migraines, colds, minor infections and an acute flare-up of irritable bowel syndrome.

Often it can feel very unfair that stress-related symptoms are held at bay when the pressure is really on and then ruin the holiday time you've been looking forward to as a reward. However, the pattern makes a great deal of sense once you understand how the body responds to stress by activating the part of the nervous system that puts the body on chemical 'high alert'. This involves a series of intricate processes that include the secretion of the stress hormones adrenalin and cortisol. The biochemical changes that take place in the body at this point allow it to rise to all sorts of stressful challenges and yet this can only be short term. As soon as the pressure is off and relaxation kicks in, the body is no longer on a chemical high of stress hormones and it's partly the coming down from these that can produce the symptoms of what we now call leisure sickness.

Potential symptoms are immensely varied and can include any of the following:

- **Tension headaches**
- **Lack of appetite**
- **Visual disturbance, nausea and migraine headaches**
- **Diarrhoea and/or constipation**
- **Minor, low-grade infections, such as a cold**
- **Fatigue and general listlessness**
- **Poor depth and quality of sleep pattern**

practical self-help

❧ If you have a holiday coming up, and you've recently been under pressure, make a deliberate effort to relax before you go away. This way, if a reaction is going to take place, you've got a chance to recover from it before you begin your holiday.

❧ Arrange the itinery for your holiday in such a way that you allow yourself at least a few days to unwind at the beginning.

❧ Treat yourself to a full body or neck and shoulder massage, especially if you have a history of tension headaches or have endured a long-haul flight.

❧ Put relaxing and rebalancing aromatherapy oils in your bathwater, massage blend, or vaporiser. These can be bought ready-blended, or you can put together a mix of your own using lavender, ylang ylang, chamomile, neroli or clary sage.

❧ Regular exercise is invaluable for helping the body burn off excess adrenalin and relax as it will encourage the body to produce the feel-good chemicals called endorphins.

TYPE OF LEISURE SICKNESS	GENERAL SYMPTOMS	WORSE FROM	BETTER FOR	REMEDY NAME
Inability to switch off at night with tense, aching muscles	- Tosses and turns all night in an effort to find a comfortable position in bed - Problems may be exaggerated by a long-haul flight or an unusual amount of physical activity	- At night - Being touched	- Resting with the head at a slightly lower angle than the body	**Arnica**
Short-fused, tense and grumpy with difficulty in getting into holiday mood	- Especially helpful for those who don't know what to do with themselves when they are away from the focus of work - Tension headaches and constipation are both likely to be linked to feeling incredibly tense	- Coffee - Alcohol - Smoking - Lack of sleep - Excessive levels of mental stress - Early in the morning	- Sound sleep - Peace and quiet - Getting the bowels moving - Later in the day	**Nux vomica**
Headaches linked to lack of sleep and low-grade dehydration	- Although the body knows it's on holiday, the mind refuses to switch off from business at night - Poor-quality sleep with headaches and a tendency for the scalp to feel tender and sensitive	- Lack of fluid - Becoming overheated - The slightest movement - Light touch	- Keeping as still as possible - Rest - Long, cold drinks - Sweating	**Bryonia**
Constipation on holiday as a result of the change in routine	- Digestive uneasiness on holiday with lots of rumbling, gurgling and bloating of the belly	- Tight clothes - High fibre foods - In the late afternoon - Becoming chilled - Boredom	- Moderate warmth - Warm drinks - Taking gentle exercise	**Lycopodium**
Cold sores and headaches that come on in hot, sunny weather	- Generally reacts very badly to being in hot, bright climates - Fluid retention, headaches and symptoms of sensitive skin all become noticeable - Lethargic, irritable and withdrawn when feeling unwell on holiday	- Getting hot and bothered - Making any physical effort - Getting overexcited	- Contact with fresh, cool air - Skipping meals - Breaking into a sweat - Cool bathing - Gentle exercise in cool conditions	**Natrum mur**

homesickness in kids

Children often feel homesick if going away is a relatively new experience for them. It can come on at any stage of the holiday and is most likely to affect those who thrive on structure and routine and who are easily thrown by the unexpected or unfamiliar. Common symptoms may include any of the following:

- **Weepiness and clinginess**
- **Disturbed sleep pattern**
- **Anxious or panicky behaviour**
- **Lack of appetite**
- **Bedwetting**
- **Emotional withdrawal and/or lack of interest in what others are involved in**

The good news is that there's a great deal of complementary support that can give your child the emotional boost needed in order to relax into the holiday experience and begin having fun.

practical self-help

❧ Pangs of homesickness are far less likely if your child is prepared beforehand for what they might expect. Show them photographs of your holiday destination and the accommodation and talk over your plans with them so they know what you will all be doing once you get there.

❧ Take a few of your child's favourite toys with you so that they have a sense of some continuity and familiarity in a new place.

❧ Children over the age of seven who become fretful and anxious when away from home may respond very well to Rescue Remedy. Dilute a couple of drops in a small glass of still mineral water and let your child take a sip or two whenever they are feeling wobbly or distressed.

❧ It may be helpful to stick to a predictable routine of activities for the first few days of a holiday so that your child establishes a sense of security. This is especially important for any child who gets upset by the unknown or surprising.

TYPE OF HOMESICKNESS	GENERAL SYMPTOMS	WORSE FROM	BETTER FOR	REMEDY NAME
Swift changes of mood from laughing to crying in a moment	- Weeping bouts descend out of the blue - Sighs continually or prone to hiccups after a particularly long or severe weepy episode - Although feeling queasy when distressed, having something small to eat relieves the nausea	- Emotional upset - Becoming chilled - Sitting and thinking about being upset	- Warmth - Eating - Distraction	**Ignatia**
Silent sadness with no desire to join in with others	- Antisocial with a real dislike of being the focus of sympathy and attention - Won't cry in front of others, but waits until alone	- Sunny, hot weather - Stuffy rooms - Being hugged - Becoming overexcited	- Fresh, cool air - Skipping meals - Gentle exercise	**Natrum mur**
Clingy, weepy and in need of attention	- Weepy at the drop of a hat with incredibly changeable moods - Shy in new places but responds very well to company and distraction - Feels much brighter and happier after a good cry with lots of sympathy being offered	- During the night - Becoming overheated - Lack of attention - Resting	- Fresh, cool air - Lots of sympathy	**Pulsatilla**
Panicky and fearful especially at night	- Lots of anxious outbursts with the possibility of night terrors - Child is overwrought and demands that something must be done to make them feel better - Symptoms develop abruptly and with great severity	- During the night - Exposure to cold winds - Getting too hot	- Unbroken sleep - Fresh air	**Aconite**

homeopathy

●

travel or motion sickness

Travel or motion sickness can ruin a journey by car, sea or plane as I know from personal experience. Although limited in its time span, the symptoms can get very intense and may include any combination of the following:

- **Nausea**
- **Recurrent episodes of vomiting and retching**
- **Dizziness**
- **A general sense of distress and disorientation**

practical self-help

❧ Discourage children from reading or generally looking down on a journey, especially if they are in a car for a long time, as this aggravates nausea and vomiting. Instead, encourage them to look out of the window at the horizon.

❧ Make sure there's an adequate supply of fresh air on a journey so, when travelling by car, keep windows slightly open and regularly go up on deck when travelling by boat.

❧ On long journeys play games with children in order to distract them and prevent boredom and frustration from making travel sickness an even bigger misery.

❧ Give children something light and easily digestible to eat before setting off on a journey as low blood sugar levels can aggravate nausea and vomiting.

❧ Avoid wearing perfume on a journey if you know you're going to be in a warm, enclosed space as strong smells can make nausea and vomiting even worse.

❧ Wear a simple acupressure device on the wrist to relieve nausea and queasiness. These can be bought from all high street chemists.

❧ Have a flask of ginger tea to hand to soothe an upset, queasy stomach.

N.B. It can be quite difficult to differentiate between the remedies given in the opposite table and therefore this is one of the few situations where it can be helpful to use a combination formula of homeopathic remedies. This type of product will include four or five common homeopathic remedies prescribed for travel sickness in a single tablet. While this is a rather unorthodox solution from a classical homeopathic perspective, which as a rule advocates the use of single remedy that covers all of the major symptoms, a complex formula can be a useful stopgap where selecting the correct remedy is genuinely challenging. You can buy these formulas in most high-street pharmacies.

TYPE OF TRAVEL SICKNESS	GENERAL SYMPTOMS	WORSE FROM	BETTER FOR	REMEDY NAME
Travel sickness with great difficulty raising vomit	- Irritable and bad-tempered when feeling sick - Feels much better as soon as they have thrown up - Shaky and chilly with headache that lodges at the back of the head	- Strong smells e.g. coffee and tobacco - Becoming chilled - Tight clothes	- After a nap - Peace and quiet - Resting	**Nux vomica**
Motion sickness brought on by having too little (or nothing) to eat before a journey	- Aversion to cool, fresh air on the head and face - Giddy with headache and nausea and feels fearful and anxious - Vomits up bile because the stomach is empty	- Motion - Getting upset and angry - Becoming chilled - Tight clothes	- Contact with comfortably warm air	**Petroleum**
Travel sickness with faintness and chill	- Headache and severe gagging and retching with unpleasant sensation of excess mucus in the mouth - Extreme sensitivity to any strong smell that makes sickness more intense	- Becoming chilled - Jarring movement - Bending forward - Making physical effort - Lack of rest	- Rest - Sleep	**Cocculus**
Motion sickness with drenching sweats on being sick	- Sickness and nausea are worse for even the slightest movement - Nasty sinking feeling in the stomach - General sense of disorientation and a specific sense of pressure around the head	- Opening or moving the eyes - Extreme variations in temperature	- Cool compresses applied to the face - Loosening clothes around the belly - After vomiting - Contact with cool air	**Tabaccum**

homeopathy

175

mild sunburn

Unfortunately, it's all too easy to get mildly sunburnt on the first couple of days of your holiday but, in a hot climate, being in the sun around the middle of the day without adequate protection can be a recipe for disaster. Symptoms can vary in intensity but may include any of the following:

- **Red, hot, flushed skin on unprotected areas**
- **Headache**
- **Slight dizziness**
- **Nausea**
- **Feeling feverish**

practical self-help

❦ Prevention is definitely the best policy. Make sure you use high factor suncreams and sunblocks, especially on vulnerable areas like the neck (especially at the nape), face, chest, arms and back.

❦ If you know you're going to be outside between mid-day and 3p.m., wear a hat to protect you from too much direct sun on the head and scalp.

❦ If, in spite of sensible precautions, you have sustained some patches of mild sunburn, apply soothing Urtica urens cream to the affected areas as it helps take the stinging and smarting out of minor burns of any kind.

❦ If the skin is flushed and sore, a cool aloe vera gel can take the heat out of the skin.

CAUTION!

IF ANY OF THE FOLLOWING OCCUR, GET EMERGENCY MEDICAL ASSISTANCE:

- Drowsiness
- Violent headache
- Vomiting
- A fever that has risen above 39–40°C/103°F
- Breathing difficulties
- Very rapid pulse

TYPE OF SUNBURN	GENERAL SYMPTOMS	WORSE FROM	BETTER FOR	REMEDY NAME
Sunburn with flushed, itchy skin	- Sudden onset of symptoms after exposure to sun - Throbbing headache with pains that are eased by contact with cool, fresh air but made worse by contact with an ice pack	- Bending the head backwards - Warmth directed at the head - Movement	- Resting with the head propped up rather than flat - Cool surroundings	**Glonoin**
Sunburn with bright red, dry skin	- Rapidly developing, burning heat in localised patches of skin that have been overexposed to sunlight - Headache with throbbing in temples	- Becoming chilled - Lack of perspiration - Noise	- Bending the head backwards - Light covering - Rest	**Belladonna**
Sunburn with exhaustion from mild dehydration	- Sunburn with a cold sensation in the body and heat in the head - Generally feels much better for contact with cool air	- Becoming chilled - Restrictive clothing - Lack of fluids	- Lying with the feet slightly elevated - Being fanned - Cold drinks	**Carbo veg**

homeopathy

●

177

9 | homeopathy for mother and baby

Homeopathy has an impeccable record when it comes to treating the problems that often crop up during pregnancy or following childbirth. For babies, it very effectively deals with the distress of everyday problems such as teething or baby colic and, as a result, newborns tend to sleep and feed better, while parents can heave a huge sigh of relief. It is also important to stress that there have been no reported instances of adverse reactions to homeopathic treatment used in pregnancy.

The following self-help is as flexible as it needs to be for each individual case. Some mothers are confident to use occasional doses of self-prescribed remedies, while others are happier to consult a homeopathic practitioner first. In order to make this decision easier, I have highlighted the symptoms in this chapter that are sure signs when the situation would benefit from professional care.

Crushing tablets is usually the best and safest method of giving remedies to babies and small children: crush the tablet between two teaspoons and rub a little of the fine powder between your child's gum and cheek. However, older children should have no problems chewing the tablets as they taste pleasantly sweet.

morning, evening and all-day sickness

The heading for this section has been deliberately expanded to account for the persistent sort of nausea and vomiting that can affect unlucky mothers all day long. Fortunately, however, it's also possible to feel nothing more than a vague feeling of queasiness and the odd bout of indigestion over the first three months; it really seems to be a lottery.

The good news is that whatever sort of sickness you experience in pregnancy, there is a homeopathic solution to the problem. In addition, you have a range of practical self-help measures that may in themselves be enough to deal with the odd, mild episode of nausea.

practical self-help

❧ If sickness really is a morning affair, get into the habit of keeping some biscuits and water close to hand in the bedroom and ideally within easy reach. As soon as you sit up in bed in the morning, have a few sips of water and a plain biscuit as an empty stomach can make the nausea more intense. Make sure you then get out of bed slowly as dizziness is likely to make the queasiness worse.

❧ Eat something small and easily digestible every couple of hours or so as blood sugar levels have a tendency to become very erratic in pregnancy and this can trigger dizziness, severe nausea, disorientation, mood swings and/or problems with concentration. As every pregnant woman knows all these can be frequent occurrences in pregnancy anyway, and so avoid coffee and any food with a high fat yield or that's laced with white sugar and opt instead for foods that guarantee a sustained energy release.

❧ Choose foods that are easily digestible and remember that the cooking method is as significant as the nutritional value of the ingredients. Stir-frying, poaching, steaming or baking are all healthy but avoid deep or shallow-frying, roasting and boiling like the plague as their cooking smells alone are often enough to get a stomach turning.

❧ During pregnancy the taste for coffee, tea, cigarettes and alcohol often disappears overnight. This is very convenient as they all have significant health drawbacks for mother and baby in pregnancy. These are well documented, apart from maybe tea which can irritate the lining of the stomach and make queasiness worse.

❧ If you find that dairy foods really set your stomach churning, make sure that you are getting enough calcium from non-dairy sources, such as green leafy vegetables, whole grains and almonds. Vegetarians also need to watch that iron levels are topped up through eating regular portions of pulses, nuts and seeds.

❧ Morning sickness can sometimes be linked to an unspoken anxiety about being pregnant and this can happen when pregnancy has either happened as a surprise, or turned out to be quite a difficult process. Pregnancy is a time of huge hormonal shifts and this can give unexpected emotions a chance to rise to the surface. If this should happen, it's very important to appreciate that it is far from uncommon and there is no reason to feel alarmed. Of course, if the pregnancy wasn't planned, it could be helpful for you to talk through the difficult emotions so that you feel reassured.

CAUTION!

IF ANY OF THE FOLLOWING OCCUR, CONSULT YOUR DOCTOR:

- Morning sickness that makes it very difficult to keep fluids down
- Nausea and vomiting that are not improved by any self-help measures
- Severe, persistent morning or all day sickness that gets worse as time goes by

TYPE OF MORNING SICKNESS	GENERAL SYMPTOMS	WORSE FROM	BETTER FOR	REMEDY NAME
Constant bad nausea that is not relieved for being sick	- Hot or cold, clammy sweat with sickness - Lots of empty retching - Nausea isn't relieved by eating and feels more intense and distressing for making even the slightest movement	- Stooping - Strong smells - Being sick	- Keeping as still as possible - Rest - Contact with cool, fresh air	**Ipecac**
Sickness and nausea that's especially intense and distressing in the morning	- Very sensitive to cooking smells that can cause retching - Unpleasant dizzy sensation with persistent headache - Sour or tart flavours appeal most when hungry - Nausea is temporarily relieved by eating	- On waking - Becoming chilled - Thinking of food - Emotional demands	- Fresh air - Keeping blood sugar levels stable - Resting in a comfortably warm bed	**Sepia**
Morning sickness with a huge sense of relief after being sick	- Although it's a massive relief once it has happened, the act of being sick can be difficult with lots of gagging and retching - Symptoms are at their most intense on waking	- Coffee and other stimulants - Spicy foods - Mental and emotional stress - Being deprived of sound sleep	- Peace and quiet - Lying down - Sound sleep - Rest - As the day goes on	**Nux vomica**
Morning sickness that continues well into the evening	- Although feeling generally chilly, warm, stuffy rooms make nausea much more distressing - Hypersensitivity to fatty foods that immediately cause nausea and 'repeating' for a long time after they have been eaten	- Resting - Warmth - Mornings and evenings	- Contact with fresh, cool air - Splashing the face with cool water - After a good cry - Lots of sympathy and attention	**Pulsatilla**

homeopathy

heartburn

Heartburn is very common during the last three to four months of pregnancy. The problem emerges partly as a result of the pressure that is exerted on the stomach by the developing foetus (after all, there's limited room in there) and partly due to the muscle that shuts off the upper part of the stomach from the gullet. If it relaxes, digestive juices tend to wash up into the throat. Symptoms can vary in severity and frequency and may include any of the following:

- **'Repeating' of food eaten hours earlier, especially when burping**
- **A periodical burning, acid sensation that rises into the gullet**
- **A persistent or intermittent nasty taste in the mouth**
- **A nagging burning sensation that lodges in the stomach and/or centre of the chest**

If you have no previous history of heartburn the chances are that, after the birth of your baby, the problem will resolve itself. However, any of the following can be combined safely in a complementary way with other strategies suggested by your doctor or obstetrician.

practical self-help

❧ Keep meals as small, light and easily digestible as possible, especially in the last three to four months of your pregnancy when you are likely to gain a significant amount of weight. During this time, your appetite should naturally incline towards this kind of food and so vegetable soups, grilled or poached fish, poultry, lightly cooked vegetable stir-fries and fruit will greatly appeal.

❧ If you have a taste for muesli but find it triggers heartburn symptoms, soak the cereal in milk, fruit juice or water overnight as it allows the starches to be broken down into sugars, which are more easily digested. If this still doesn't solve the problem, consider switching to porridge which is soothing to the stomach while also being excellent for the circulatory system.

❧ If you notice that heartburn symptoms are especially bad at night when lying in bed, don't eat your evening meal too late (anything after 7p.m. is unwise if you go to bed early). Digestion works more slower and therefore food cannot be broken down as efficiently as it can during waking hours. Full-fat cheeses and red meat are difficult for the stomach to digest even at the best of times and therefore it's best to eat small, nutritious meals at regular intervals throughout the day and to have a small, light snack if you are hungry in the evening.

❧ Prop yourself up in bed with two or three pillows under your head but avoid this if you suffer from swollen or puffy ankles.

TYPE OF HEARTBURN	GENERAL SYMPTOMS	WORSE FROM	BETTER FOR	REMEDY NAME
Heartburn that comes on straight after eating	- A strong aversion to drinking cold water; even the sight of it causes nausea and sickness - Empty, hollow feeling in stomach with digestive uneasiness	- Lack of fluid - Lying flat - Warm food and drink - Eating salty food	- Resting - Sympathetic company and being distracted	**Phosphorus**
Heartburn with acid that washes into the throat	- Burning discomfort in the stomach that can extend all the way up into the throat - Lots of burping with a small amount of acid coming up each time - Can't eat much at a single sitting	- Eating too much in one go - Too many high-fibre foods - Feeling stressed and anxious	- Taking a gentle stroll in the fresh air - Loosening clothing - Eating small amounts often	**Lycopodium**
Heartburn that's relieved by taking small sips of a warm drink	- Feels generally uncomfortable, restless and anxious during the night - Burning and acidity with heartburn and a tendency to diarrhoea	- Cold food and drink - When alone - In the early hours of the morning	- Lying propped up on two or three pillows - Feeling comfortably warm - Company	**Arsenicum album**
Heartburn from too much rich food	- Heartburn and queasiness are accompanied by a dry mouth with no thirst - Lots of burping and 'repeating' of foods eaten hours before - Noticeably tearful and weepy when feeling unwell	- Stuffy, airless rooms - Warm drinks - Getting too hot in bed at night - When resting	- Gentle exercise in the fresh air - Well ventilated rooms - After a good cry	**Pulsatilla**

homeopathy

homeopathy in labour and childbirth

Homeopathy, in common with other complementary therapies such as use of TEMS machine and aromatherapy, can have an extremely practical and positive role to play in childbirth and delivery, as well as providing essential support in speeding up recovery after the birth. During each stage of the labour a homeopathic remedy can be used to reduce feelings of anxiety and panic, give a boost to flagging energy levels and take the edge off the pain so it is far more manageable.

Although some midwifery courses offer introductory sessions in the use of alternative and complementary medicines, it can still be difficult to obtain the services of a midwife who is fully qualified in homeopathy. As a result, it may be more satisfactory to ask your homeopath (if you already have one) if they would be willing to attend the birth, with the consent of the midwife and/or obsetrician who will be delivering your baby. Alternatively, but not so satisfactorily, you can use a kit, designed to give you a range of some of the most commonly indicated remedies in labour and childbirth. If your partner is happy to select the appropriate remedy for you at each stage of the labour, it would be extremely valuable (and really rather essential) for you both to have a session with your homeopathic practitioner beforehand.

The following table includes the most commonly indicated remedies used in straightforward labours but these are here to give a general picture of the potential application of each remedy, rather than to encourage self-prescribing.

TYPE OF LABOUR	GENERAL SYMPTOMS	WORSE FROM	BETTER FOR	REMEDY NAME
Frantic, and frustrated with labour pains that are slow to progress	- Labour pains feel unbearable to the point that it is tempting to give up - Cervix is slow to dilate with severe contractions that lodge in the back	- Getting too hot - Contact with cool air	- Sweating - Cooling off when overheated - Moderate, stable temperatures	**Chamomilla**
Labour pains with regular episodes of vomiting as contractions occur	- Impatient, irritable and abusive in labour - Contractions lead to bruised, exhausting pains - Because of the amount of straining with each contraction, there is a sensation as though about to pass a stool	- Becoming chilled - Being touched	- Quiet surroundings - Warmth	**Nux vomica**

TYPE OF LABOUR	GENERAL SYMPTOMS	WORSE FROM	BETTER FOR	REMEDY NAME
Terror-stricken and panicky at second stage of labour	- Extreme restlessness and intolerance of labour pains - Can be especially useful when labour is violent and fast	- Being examined - Extreme change of temperature	- Fresh air - Being uncovered	**Aconite**
Weak labour pains with slow dilation of cervix	- Labour is long, slow and very exhausting - Pains are severe and seem to fly about in all directions - Trembles and shivers in pain but craves fresh air, although feeling chilly	- Becoming chilled - Contact with cold air - Exhaustion	- Contact with fresh air	**Caulophyllum**
Slow to start labour, or one that keeps stopping and starting	- Pains are weak and only occur intermittently - General sense of distress is intensified by overheated, badly ventilated environment - Some weepiness	- Absence of sympathy - Having to keep still - Lack of fresh air	- Cool compresses to the head - Being able to move around - Sympathy and encouragement	**Pulsatilla**
Labour pains that settle in the back and radiate to the buttocks	- Pain of contractions is relieved by applying firm pressure to, or massaging the back - It also helps to assume a squatting position with elbows supported on the knees	- Becoming chilled - Being uncovered	- Warmth - Massage - Firm pressure to painful area	**Kali carb**
Rapid exhaustion in first stage of labour with fear of not being able to cope	- Contraction pains are heavy and exhausting and often lodge in the back - Contractions stop on, or after, examination - Legs feel weak and wobbly as a result of the effort of coping with the contractions	- Becoming overheated - Becoming chilled - Anxiety	- Sweating - Being able to move about - Contact with fresh air	**Gelsemium**

homeopathy

185

recovery after the birth

This is an area where homeopathy really comes into its own as it can help new mothers to a sense of emotional and physical equilibrium in no time at all. This is always desirable, but especially for mums who already have a young child or two waiting impatiently for them and the new baby to arrive back home.

Homeopathic prescribing can also be hugely helpful for mothers who found that their experience of giving birth was quite different to the delivery that they expected. Unfortunately, this can often happen during the first experience of childbirth if events take an unexpected turn and derail the detailed birth plan you have drawn up in advance. If the medical assistance you require is something you had initially thought of as undesirable and planned to avoid, this can understandably lead to negative feelings after the birth. Anger, a profound sense of disappointment, resentment, guilt and a painful sense of failure can all obstruct the new mother's natural excitement and exhilaration. Therefore, effective homeopathic prescribing in the days following delivery can be of vital assistance not only in smoothing out emotional upsets but in gently and speedily relieving the pain and discomfort of an episiotomy and vaginal bruising.

practical self-help

❧ Bathing in a bidet that contains a diluted solution of Calendula tincture (one part tincture to ten parts warm water) can speed up the healing of traumatised areas with astonishing speed.

❧ If stitches are especially tender and painful, bathing in a combined solution of Calendula and Hypericum tincture (marketed as 'Hypercal') is extremely effective. calendula, made from marigold, is a natural antiseptic that encourages damaged tissue to heal and Hypericum is particularly good for soothing and relieving pain in areas that are especially rich in nerve endings.

❧ If regular bathing in a bidet isn't an option, a diluted solution of either tincture may be used to moisten a sanitary pad that can be changed at regular intervals in order to soothe and heal the perineum.

❧ If bathing in Calendula or Hypercal tincture feels soothing, the gentle healing effect can be enhanced by applying either formula at regular intervals in a cream form to the traumatised areas.

TYPE OF TRAUMA	GENERAL SYMPTOMS	WORSE FROM	BETTER FOR	REMEDY NAME
Internal and external bruising following delivery	- This is the all-purpose remedy for the physical and emotional shock that can follow even the most textbook birth – it promotes effective healing of localised bruising and reduces tenderness, aching and swelling	- Touch - Being examined - Jarring movement	- Resting	**Arnica**
Deep bruising and aching that's not totally resolved by Arnica	- General feelings of tiredness and exhaustion with squeezing, throbbing pains - This remedy may be especially helpful after a forceps or venteuse delivery	- Touch - Getting warm or overheated in bed - Bathing	- Cool compresses - Continuous gentle movement	**Bellis perennis**
Residual pains that are left after an epidural or episiotomy	- Shooting, tearing pains continue for longer than expected in a stitched episiotomy or tear - Persistent back pain may date from having an epidural with shooting pains radiating from the point of insertion	- Jarring - Sudden movement - Exertion of any kind	- Massage - Relaxing on the stomach	**Hypericum**
Sharp, stinging pains with emotional distress that follow a Caesarean	- This remedy works almost like magic after an unwanted hi-tech birth - Stitching, stinging pains feel unbearably sensitive, while emotional distress takes the form of guilt, resentment and unexpressed anger at being cheated out of a natural birth	- Pressure from clothes or bed covers - Passing water - At night - Emotional stress	- Warmth - Resting	**Staphysagria**

homeopathy

re-establishing emotional balance (baby blues)

Getting back on track physically and emotionally after the birth can be something of a rollercoaster. The highs and lows can be equally intense and, provided they are short-lived, they are part and parcel of normal motherhood. After all, broken sleep, the demands of regular feeds and getting to know a new baby are going to be a pretty big challenge at first for anyone!

However, if any of the following become a persistent or noticeable feature of life, it's definitely worth getting some extra professional support from an alternative therapist or conventional health visitor or family doctor:

- **A feeling of being swamped and unable to cope with minor, day-to-day tasks**
- **Involuntary, frequent, long-lasting episodes of weepiness that descend without any warning**
- **Uncharacteristic feelings of depression, indifference, emotional numbness or lack of motivation**
- **Feelings of negativity or despair on waking**
- **Severe, persistent anxiety about your own health or that of your baby**
- **A profound sense of physical, mental and emotional exhaustion that isn't relieved by periods of rest or relaxation**

Most mothers will be familiar with some of these emotions as, in the short term, they are quite natural reactions to adjusting to the emotional and physical demands that motherhood brings in its wake. However, if the 'blues' become a regular feature of life, or if they become more rather than less intense as time goes by, it's time to look for extra help and support.

Anyone who is uneasy about choosing conventional antidepressants as their first port of call and who would like to try an alternative source of treatment at least first, may prefer to consult a western medical herbalist or homeopath. If high stress levels are a contributory factor, extra practical support can be provided in the form of aromatherapy or reflexology.

practical self-help

It's very important to acknowledge uncomfortable feelings, rather than taking refuge in a stiff upper lip approach, as suppressed emotions very rarely go away and often create more long-term difficulties by giving rise to other fears and phobias that seem to have no rationale behind them. Unacknowledged emotions, if they remain buried for long enough, can also be a co-factor in developing muscle aches and pains, digestive problems, tension headaches, migraines or any other condition that falls into the general category of 'stress related'.

❧ Talk about how you're feeling with someone you can trust – especially if you're harbouring negative, painful and unresolved feelings about your experience of pregnancy and/or childbirth that are preventing you from bonding successfully with your baby. If you like the idea of talking openly to someone who is able to take an objective perspective on your situation then a trained counsellor might be your best choice.

❧ Keep in contact with some of the other mothers you have formed a bond with at ante-natal or relaxation classes. It can be incredibly reassuring to talk frankly with someone you like who is going through a similar experience.

❧ If you know you're holding a lot of tension in your neck and shoulders – a clenched jaw is a very big giveaway – book yourself a regular neck and shoulder massage with soothing, stress-busting aromatherapy oils. Not only will this give your body the pampering it's probably crying out for but it will also give you back a sense of doing something positive for yourself.

❧ Although tempting, avoid taking refuge in the odd additional glass of wine or extra large gin and tonic when feeling low. Alcohol is a powerful depressant and therefore feelings of anxiety and/or depression are far more likely to surface after a drink or two too many. Opt instead for fruit-based drinks with energy-balancing herbal ingredients such as ginseng – many of them contain ginger extract and will therefore benefit your digestion as well. N.B. If you are breastfeeding, check with your pharmacist that any herbs you are considering taking are safe in the situation.

CAUTION!

IF ANY OF THE FOLLOWING OCCUR, CONSULT YOUR DOCTOR:

- Emotional numbness that alternates with episodes of violent anger
- Depressive feelings that don't respond to self-help measures
- Thoughts of self-harm or harm to your baby
- A sense of persistent detachment or of losing touch with reality

Homeopathic Support Table overleaf

TYPE OF BABY BLUES	GENERAL SYMPTOMS	WORSE FROM	BETTER FOR	REMEDY NAME
Indifferent and irritable and finding it hard to bond with your baby	- Pervading sense of being unable to cope with a fear of going out of control - Profound sense of mental, emotional and physical exhaustion - Weepy, withdrawn and despondent with an absent libido	- Emotional demands or pressure - Rest - Being touched - Sympathy and attention	- Brisk, aerobic exercise in the fresh air - Eating small amounts often - After a sound sleep	**Sepia**
Severe, abruptly changing mood swings with bouts of uncontrollable weepiness	- This remedy is helpful in the days following childbirth when moods can rollercoaster dramatically - Overwhelming sense of loss at the fact that physical separation has occurred	- Alcohol - Stimulants (such as caffeine) - Becoming chilled	- Warmth - Eating small amounts often - Distraction	**Ignatia**
Withdrawn and depressed with an inability to cry	- Depressive, low mood that's worse for sympathetic company and being the focus of attention - Although very sensitive and easily hurt, the surface appearance is one of reservation and a stiff upper lip	- Company - Being seen to cry - Being hugged	- Being given some breathing space - Rest - Skipping meals - Contact with cool, fresh air	**Natrum mur**
Depression that stems from a sense of suppressed guilt, pain or resentment about the birth	- This is often needed when a mother is left feeling physically traumatised or violated due to receiving undesired medical intervention during the birth - Depression is common when these feelings of anger turn inwards instead of being talked about and resolved	- Sensual contact - Touch - Becoming angry over something of minor importance	- Resting - Comfort eating - Warmth	**Staphisagria**

teething

Teething is almost as much of a lottery for babies as morning sickness is for mothers-to-be: some seem to waltz through it with hardly a twinge, while others find the whole process extremely distressing. Generally speaking, problems don't start during the first year as associated symptoms are often nothing more dramatic than wanting to chew on something hard, as well as a tendency to extravagant drooling. However, once the next phase gets under way (usually any time between the age of one and three), more difficult and distressing symptoms can be quite common. These may include any of the following:

- **Heat, swelling and inflammation of the affected gums**
- **Loose stools**
- **Hypersensitivity and tenderness where the teeth are breaking through**
- **Swelling and redness of the cheek on the affected side**
- **Loss of appetite**
- **Lethargy and listlessness**
- **Emotional short fuse and weepiness at the least thing**

In this situation, conventional medicine offers sedative formulations and yet many parents are uneasy about becoming too reliant on these, using them only when they are desperate to get some rest for themselves and their toddler. However, practical, alternative therapies can render the use of conventional sedatives unnecessary and this includes any of the following.

practical self-help

❧ Sore, inflamed gums can be temporarily relieved by the application of firm pressure. Rub the painful area or encourage older toddlers to bite on something hard – you can buy teething biscuits with a ribbon attached (this is an important safety feature, as babies always have to be watched when chewing anything in order to guard against the risk of choking).

❧ Cool objects are good at relieving the discomfort of teething. Try a teething ring that can be cooled from the inside by filling a cavity with cold water, or keep a fresh, scrupulously clean flannel in the fridge that can be taken out and sucked on.

❧ Rub a cool infusion of chamomile tea into the painful area or paint the outside of the affected, swollen cheek with an aromatherapy oil mixture. The simplest formula is made by adding five drops of Roman chamomile essential oil to 50ml (1³/4fl oz) jojoba oil. Apply this to the sore cheek up to three or four times daily, depending on demand.

Homeopathic Support Table overleaf

TYPE OF TEETHING PROBLEM	GENERAL SYMPTOMS	WORSE FROM	BETTER FOR	REMEDY NAME
Teething pains that go into overdrive at night	- Teething baby often goes to sleep seeming fine, only to wake in a state of huge distress with teething pains that seem to be intolerable	- Becoming overheated - Becoming chilled - Waking from sleep in pain	- Moderate warmth - Sound sleep	**Aconite**
Frantic howling and distress with teething	- Baby is noticeably flushed when upset and in pain, with one cheek often redder than the other - Colicky pains and loose stools with teething	- Becoming overheated - Becoming chilled - During the night	- Cool compresses applied to sensitive area - Gentle rocking - Moderately warm surroundings	**Chamomilla**
Noticeably delayed teething pattern	- Teething causes a lot of distress and discomfort - Walking and talking may also occur later than expected - Babies and toddlers who do well with this remedy are likely to be pale, chilly, on the thin side and with poor energy levels and sluggish resistance to minor infections	- Physical effort - Exhaustion	- Having a warm bath - Rest - Moderate warmth	**Calc phos**

CAUTION!

IF ANY OF THE FOLLOWING OCCUR, CONSULT YOUR DOCTOR:

- **Well-established or severe catarrhal (blocked/runny nose, chesty cough and/or ear problems) and/or digestive upsets that are associated with teething**
- **If pain and distress aren't promptly and substantially relieved by self-help measures**
- **General signs of uncharacteristic distress, listlessness or lethargy with teething symptoms**

baby colic

I have seen many parents at their wits' end when their new baby develops severe symptoms of colic for, while not a cause for concern in itself, baby colic can cause extreme distress and disruption to a young family. The symptoms are pretty easy to spot and may include any of the following:

- **Sharp pains in the stomach and belly that often cause the baby to draw his or her knees up to the chest – this may be done as an instinctive reflex to apply firm pressure to the painful area**
- **Lots of wailing and screaming with a tendency for the face to get flushed up**
- **Symptoms come on swiftly after feeding, or are especially severe as the day goes on or in the evening**
- **Signs of excess gas or constipation**
- **Symptoms characteristically set in any time after birth and may last for approximately three months or so**

practical self-help

❧ If you have a colicky baby and you are breastfeeding, eliminate strong tea, coffee, alcohol, raw onions, raw peppers, cabbage, cauliflower, sprouts, cucumber, citrus fruits and spicy foods such as chillies and curries from your diet as these have a reputation for aggravating the problem.

❧ When breastfeeding, always ensure that your baby is well latched on to your nipple to avoid them sucking in extra air.

❧ When bottle-feeding, always check that the teat on your baby's bottle is the right size. If it isn't, there's a risk that too much air will be swallowed at the same time as the milk and, as you can imagine, if this goes on at each feed trapped wind will become an additional complication.

❧ If you are using formula, check that it has been made up correctly as the wailing could also be triggered by thirst; from too concentrated a formula that is too high in salt, or from hunger pangs that are a result of the formula being too dilute.

❧ Soothing a constantly colicky baby can really wear you down as nothing you do seems to help at all. In this situation, hand your baby over to someone else in your household who is feeling less stressed as babies often pick up on feelings and respond accordingly. This is a helpful damage-limitation exercise and should avoid creating a vicious circle of frustration that moves from baby to mother and back again.

❧ Applying a warm but not overly hot compress (do test it first) to your baby's abdomen can help soothe the distress of colic, especially if you soak the compress in a warm herbal infusion before applying it to the belly. Suitable stress-reducing, anti-spasmodic herbs to choose from include chamomile, linden blossom, lemon balm or hops. To make the infusion add half a teaspoon of the selected herb to 100ml (3¹/₂oz) boiling water. Leave to stand for fifteen minutes before straining and allow it to cool before use – to be extra sure, test the temperature on the back of your arm before using.

❧ Massage is always soothing and is especially good at releasing trapped wind in a baby's stomach or abdomen. Use a plain carrier oil in order to encourage your hands to move smoothly over your baby's skin and always warm the oil in your hands before applying it (never drop cool oil on the skin surface as this can feel jarring). Using gentle pressure, massage your baby's back or their abdomen, making slow, circular movements.

❧ If you suspect that constipation is contributing to problems with occasional colic in your baby, make sure that they drink plenty of fluid, particularly in hot, dry weather. Massage helps encourage regular bowel movements or, with older infants who are on solids, abdominal discomfort can be eased by adding cooked, finely mashed prunes or apricots to their food.

CAUTION!

IF ANY OF THE FOLLOWING OCCUR, CONSULT YOUR DOCTOR:

- **If you sense your baby is uncharacteristically distressed**
- **Signs of vomiting, diarrhoea and scanty flow of urine in a severely distressed baby**

TYPE OF COLIC	GENERAL SYMPTOMS	WORSE FROM	BETTER FOR	REMEDY NAME
Normally content baby becomes clingy and weepy	- Distressing bouts of colic with changeable stools – no two bowel movements look alike - Colic may have come on, or be noticeably worse for mother eating a rich, fatty diet when breastfeeding	- Hot, stuffy rooms - Heavy clothes or bedcovers - Keeping still	- Being carried outside in the fresh air - Pressure of heavy bedcovers - Keeping still	**Pulsatilla**

TYPE OF COLIC	GENERAL SYMPTOMS	WORSE FROM	BETTER FOR	REMEDY NAME
Baby can't be consoled due to the distress that colic causes	- Lots of yelling and screaming makes the baby puce in the face - Distended abdomen that isn't relieved by passing wind - Child throws offered toys to the floor in sheer frustration	- At night	- Being rocked or being taken for a short drive - Warm compresses	**Chamomilla**
Colicky pains that are soothed by firm pressure to the belly	- Baby instinctively lies on its front or pushes its fists into the belly in order to ease the pain - As the pain sets in or builds, the baby doubles up or pulls knees up to the chest	- Keeping still - Releasing pressure from abdomen	- Warmth applied to sensitive area - Movement - Release of trapped wind	**Colocythis**
Colicky pains and constipation	- Colic aggravated by breastfeeding mother eating lots of spicy foods and/or drinking lots of strong coffee - Discomfort is most noticeable when waking from an interrupted nap	- After eating - Touch - Pressure - Lack of sleep - Becoming chilled	- Rest - Sound, uninterrupted sleep - Warmth	**Nux vomica**
Colic that's noticeably more intense in the early or late afternoon	- Lots of loud rumbling and gurgling sounds with colicky pains that are triggered by each feed - The situation may unwittingly be aggravated by a breastfeeding mother eating too much fibre (e.g. wholewheat, beans and pulses)	- After each feed - Becoming overheated - Cold drinks	- Release of wind - Warm drinks - Loosening clothes around the waist	**Lycopodium**
Colic that is more intense when teething	- Distress of colic is noticeably soothed by gentle massage - Along with the pain, the infant produces a disproportionate amount of gas that travels downwards	- Tight, restrictive clothing - Cold drinks - At night - Becoming chilled	- Warmth - Firm pressure	**Mag phos**

homeopathy

195

nappy rash

This persistent problem can really blight the lives of mothers and babies so it's very important to treat the problem as early as possible in order to avoid the complication of a secondary infection taking hold. Common symptoms may include any of the following:

- **A mild or noticeably inflamed rash that covers the bottom, thighs and/or genital area**
- **In severe cases, raised, red patches get more sensitive after passing water or a bowel movement**
- **White patches inside the mouth would suggest your baby has got oral thrush, which aggravates nappy rash as it spreads through the digestive tract**

While any of the following measures may effectively clear up a mild attack of recent onset nappy rash, a well-established and/or severe episode will require professional complementary treatment to eradicate the problem.

practical self-help

> Allow as much air as possible to come into contact with the affected area in order to speed up the healing process. This is important as warm, moist conditions really aggravate the discomfort of the rash. When convenient, leave your baby's nappy off for as long as possible and be prepared for the inevitable but hopefully occasional accident!

> Avoid waterproof pants as these perpetuate the problem by trapping in moisture. Try a different variety of disposable nappies or terry towelling with liners until you discover the best and most comfortable combination.

> Dry the affected area gently but thoroughly each time after washing and make a point of changing damp or soiled nappies as promptly as possible.

> With washable nappies, make sure they are rinsed thoroughly after washing, and avoid using biological formulations of detergent due to their reputation for aggravating problems with sensitive skin.

> After each nappy change, apply Calendula cream to the sore area in order to soothe the skin and speed up the healing process but make sure that the skin is completely dry first.

TYPE OF NAPPY RASH	GENERAL SYMPTOMS	WORSE FROM	BETTER FOR	REMEDY NAME
First stage of nappy rash with rapid onset of symptoms	- Hot, bright red rash that radiates heat - Normally placid babies become very irritable and fractious when uncomfortable - If it responds well to this remedy, the rash can clear up as quickly as it emerged	- Touch - Even light pressure to the affected area - Jarring movement	- Resting - Moderate warmth	**Belladonna**
Rosy-pink-looking rash	- Rash looks shiny, puffy or raised as though fluid is trapped under the spots - Discomfort is obviously soothed by contact with cool air or water	- Being touched - Becoming heated - Contact with damp - Too hot clothes	- Taking clothing off - Contact with cool air - Gentle movement	**Apis**
Fast-developing rash that causes great distress at night	- Hot, sore spots that are obviously very sensitive after urinating - Sleep pattern is severely disturbed resulting in a cranky and drowsy baby during the day	- During and after passing water - Becoming chilled - Movement - Touch	- Comfortable warmth that doesn't overheat	**Cantharis**
Poor healing skin with nappy rash	- Moist-looking nappy rash that settles in the folds of skin around the genital area and buttocks - Discomfort is aggravated by becoming too hot	- Becoming overheated - Skin being kept damp - At night	- Exposure to fresh air	**Graphites**

cradle cap

This problem is common around the hairline and scalp and can develop any time from three months up to three years of age. It can also spread to the ears or eyebrows and looks rather like dandruff on the skin. Additional symptoms can include the following:

- **A crusty, scaly eruption on the scalp that may be white or brownish-yellow in colour**
- **Spots on the face that look like little pimples or blotches. These become more noticeable when a baby is overheated or distressed**

Any of the following measures can be effective in clearing up a recent, mild episode of cradle cap. However, if symptoms are severe or well established, you will get better results from consulting a trained homeopath as they will aim to provide a more deep-seated treatment to eradicate the underlying tendency in your baby's constitution.

practical self-help

❧ Avoid the temptation to pick off any crusts or scales that aren't loose, as this can cause bleeding, soreness and possible infection. Loose scales, however can be gently and carefully removed with a soft brush.

❧ Scales can be loosened by gently rubbing a softening oil into the affected areas of the scalp. Almond oil is excellent for the purpose as it is quite light but olive oil is good if you feel that a denser, heavier oil is called for. Leave the oil on overnight and carefully comb the scalp the following morning. This should readily detach the scales without any need for pulling or tugging. Follow this procedure by washing the scalp gently with a pH-balanced shampoo, taking great care to rinse all traces of shampoo away.

❧ Apply Calendula ointment or cream morning and evening to the scalp. Use the ointment formulation if the scales and crusts need a lot of intense moisture but avoid this if your baby is sensitive to lanolin. The cream is excellent where a lighter texture is required.

TYPE OF CRADLE CAP	GENERAL SYMPTOMS	WORSE FROM	BETTER FOR	REMEDY NAME
Cradle cap that's especially severe around the hair margin	- Very dry, flaky skin texture overall with a tendency to be cracked and chapped in high summer or mid-winter - Lips are especially dry and cracked in the corners of the mouth or in the middle of the lower lip	- Being held and comforted - Direct sunlight on the skin - Touch	- Contact with fresh, cool air - Sweating - Rubbing	**Natrum mur**
Maddeningly itchy cradle cap that triggers restlessness at night	- Baby scratches and worries at the scalp in an effort to ease the itching and irritation - Cradle cap looks thick, crusty and moist	- During the night - When in bed - Becoming chilled - Exposure to warmth	- Motion	**Rhus tox**
Cradle cap that gets worse for being covered up	- Scales look thick, like dandruff, and may have a brownish tinge - Skin has a generally dry, parched texture, with a noticeable tendency to chapping in the fold	- Where scales are covered by clothing - Becoming too warm	- Distraction - Contact with fresh air - Stable, moderate temperatures	**Lycopodium**
Scurfy cradle cap with a tendency for the head to sweat easily	- Especially suited for cradle cap that develops in chubby, chilly babies who sweat easily, especially around the head at night - All milestones, such as crawling, sitting up, and walking happen later than expected	- Washing - Extreme changes of temperature	- Cooling off without becoming chilled - Being touched	**Calc carb**

homeopathy

●

199

haemorrhoids (piles)

This medical problem can be excruciatingly painful as it causes the veins in the rectum and/or anus to become swollen, irritated and inflamed. Common symptoms can include any combination of the following:

- **Severe pain on passing a stool which persists for a considerable time afterwards**
- **Bleeding after passing a stool (with piles, the blood should be bright red in colour)**
- **Itching in the rectum and/or anus**
- **A tendency to piles is usually associated with a history of constipation or irritable bowel syndrome where there is a history of alternation between constipation and diarrhoea**
- **Possible mucus discharge during or after passing a stool**

The measures listed below can do a great deal to ease the distress of an acute flare-up of mild to moderate piles. However, for more severe or very well-established problems with this condition it is a good idea to seek treatment from an experienced homeopathic practitioner.

practical self-help

⚒ A warm bath or a cool compress can temporarily ease the itching and aching of sensitive piles.

⚒ Apply herbal creams containing Aesculus hippocastum, Aloe and Hamamelis, which are designed to reduce the inflammation and itching of haemorrhoids.

⚒ Add a handful of sea salt to a soothing warm bath.

⚒ If constipation is adding to your problems, check your fibre intake and also assess how much water you drink on a daily basis, not counting tea, coffee or alcohol. This is significant as water bulks out and softens stools, making them easier to pass.

⚒ If your lifestyle is quite sedentary, include some regular exercise into your routine. The regular rhythmic motion of brisk walking, jogging or running is known to stimulate the bowel and, if you're in any doubt about this, ask any runners that you know well how many times exercising has prompted an urgent need to 'go'.

CAUTION!

IF ANY OF THE FOLLOWING OCCUR, CONSULT YOUR DOCTOR:

- Signs of severe or persistent bleeding from the rectum
- Stools that look inexplicably dark or tarry in colour, or noticeably different in texture to what is normal
- Any change in bowel habit that can't be put down to obvious causes, such as a stomach upset, change in diet, travelling, or obvious escalation in stress levels

TYPE OF PILES	GENERAL SYMPTOMS	WORSE FROM	BETTER FOR	REMEDY NAME
Piles that are sensitive to touch and bleed very easily	- History of constipation - Piles feel full and inflamed while the rectum feels tight and narrow - Irritable and short-fused with pains that radiate up the spine	- Stress - Poor diet with lots of junk food - Painkillers	- Managing to clear the bowel - Warmth - Rest - Peace and quiet	**Nux vomica**
Piles with sharp, prickling, stinging pains	- Tense, tight feeling in piles as though they are on the point of exploding - Bleeding occurs very easily and frequently with persistent soreness after bleeding has stopped	- Jarring motion, e.g. running on a hard surface - Becoming chilled - Touch or pressure		**Hamamelis**
Piles with a sense of inactivity in the rectum	- Piles cause pains that continue long after a stool (likely to be very large, hard and impacted) has finally been passed - Excruciatingly sensitive piles react very badly to the slightest movement or light pressure	- Warmth - Moving around - Coughing	- Keeping completely still - Long, cold drinks of water - Coolness; contact with cool air and compresses	**Bryonia**
Prolapsed piles that appear at the menopause	- Sharp pains that linger for hours after passing a stool - At its height, the discomfort feels as though the rectum is packed with small, sharp sticks and splinters - Tight feeling with burning sensation in the anus	- Lying down - Standing for long periods of time - On waking	- Cool water locally applied - Uncovering so that cool fresh air can get to the painful parts - Exercise	**Aesculus**
Piles with itching after a bowel movement	- Upward-moving, stinging pains with lots of urging and straining, even when attempting to pass a soft stool	- Too much starch in the diet - Getting warm in bed - Sitting - Physical effort	- Rest - Cool bathing - Contact with fresh air	**Alumina**

homeopathy

●

0 homeopathy and children's health

Children respond decisively and positively to homeopathic prescribing for a wide range of acute ailments. I've never come across a definitive explanation for why this should be the case, but it may be linked to the way in which children's recuperative powers are especially vigorous. Considering that homeopathy appears to work by stimulating the body's capacity for self-regulation and self-healing, it makes sense that this response is very fast in children.

However, it must be stressed that there is also a flipside to this encouraging picture for while children have astonishing recuperative powers, they also have an equally dramatic capacity to go downhill very, very quickly when unwell and conditions can escalate rapidly. Always be vigilant when home prescribing for acute children's ailments and if there is any doubt that the child has moved from a state of general illness to a graver condition, lose no time in getting medical assistance. The signs and symptoms that would indicate a worsening situation are all clearly listed in the 'Caution!' section under every condition in this chapter, and show you exactly what to look out for.

stomach upsets

These are a common nuisance and can be the result of constipation, a stomach bug or eating an unwise combination and/or amount of food at a birthday party! Some acute illnesses can also include stomach upsets as an early sign and symptom of illness. Symptoms can vary in intensity and may include any combination of the following:

- **Vague pains in the stomach and/or gut**
- **Lack of appetite**
- **Vomiting and/or diarrhoea**
- **Generally feeling off-colour and lethargic**
- **Constipation**

The conventional medical advice is to keep fluid intake up and not force food on a child if they don't feel hungry. Any of the following measures can help clear up a minor stomach upset in double-quick time and all can be used safely in any combination with conventional medicine.

practical self-help

❧ Keep fluid intake at a healthy level even if your child isn't especially thirsty in order to encourage the system to flush itself out as quickly and efficiently as possible. If your child is suffering from diarrhoea and/or vomiting then this should be an even higher priority in order to prevent dehydration. Avoid overly acidic juices that can irritate an already sensitive stomach and gut and try diluted apple juice or lightly flavoured mineral waters instead.

❧ Small sips of warm peppermint or fennel tea can do a great deal to soothe the distress and discomfort of an upset stomach.

❧ If trapped wind is causing a problem gently massage your child's back or belly, depending on which feels more soothing. This can be especially comforting to children who become frightened or distressed when feeling ill.

❧ Stomach cramps can be relieved with a warm compress. Add half a teaspoonful of chamomile, lemon balm or linden blossom to 100ml boiling water. Leave to steep for 15 minutes before straining off the liquid and leaving to cool down. Soak a soft, clean cloth in this warm infusion for a few minutes, wring out and then apply to the sensitive area.

❧ Stomach upsets that are a result of constipation can be eased by drinking lots of fluids and eating lots of fresh fruit and vegetables.

CAUTION!

• If a stomach upset is accompanied by severe pain in the abdomen, vomiting and high temperature, get swift medical assistance

• Severe and/or recurrent diarrhoea that refuses to clear up should be investigated by your doctor

TYPE OF STOMACH UPSET	GENERAL SYMPTOMS	WORSE FROM	BETTER FOR	REMEDY NAME
Stomach upsets that follow over-eating	- Nausea with a feeling as though vomiting would relieve the situation - Constipation with colicky pains - Bad tempered and crotchety when feeling unwell	- Eating an unwise mixture of food and drink - Pressure or touch - Eating	- Vomiting - Passing a stool - Warmth - Rest	**Nux vomica**
Nausea and diarrhoea that come on after eating too much ice cream or fruit	- Burning pains in the stomach that are temporarily eased by taking small sips of warm drinks - Nausea and vomiting and/or diarrhoea cause anxiety and restlessness, especially at night - Exhausted, chilly and very pale when feeling ill	- Becoming chilled - When alone - Cold or iced drinks - In the dark	- Comfortably warm surroundings - Sips of a warm drink - Resting propped up on a few pillows	**Arsenicum album**
Upset stomach from eating too much fatty food	- Nausea, burping and repeating of food eaten earlier - Heavy, uneasy sensation in the stomach - Dry sensation in the mouth without thirst	- Resting - Lying down - Eating - Ices - Warm food and drink	- Cold food and drink - Gentle exercise - Being outside in the fresh air - Massage	**Pulsatilla**
Upset stomach with lots of painful trapped wind	- Feels weak, sick and exhausted with an upset stomach - Although feeling chilly, likes being fanned or having a window open - Nasty taste in the mouth when burping	- Too much rich food - Tight clothes - Getting too hot	- Burping - Contact with fresh, cool air - Resting with the feet slightly elevated	**Carbo veg**

homeopathy

205

croup

This alarming-sounding condition is not unusual in young children, especially under the age of five. In essence, it is caused by inflammation of the larynx which in adults is called laryngitis but, because children are so underdeveloped, any noticeable inflammation of this area triggers a dramatic sound called stridor. Symptoms can vary in severity and may include any combination of the following:

- **A hoarse, rasping sound that is audible on breathing in, caused by a swollen, and/or inflamed airway**
- **Discomfort in the chest**
- **A barking cough**
- **Sensitivity around the area of the throat**
- **Any of these symptoms is likely to set in or be more severe during the night**

The conventional medical approach for a mild case of croup consists of giving reassurance to lessen the fear and panic that your child is likely to be showing. Moving to a steamy atmosphere can make it easier to breathe so turning the shower on and sitting in a steamy bathroom can bring relief. However, severe cases may need a short hospital admission in order to administer steroids and oxygen and in order to reduce respiratory distress.

practical self-help

❧ If your child is fearful, panicky and tense then croup symptoms will inevitably be more severe and distressing. Speak reassuringly and calmly and stay close to your child, sitting them on your knee and stroking their back.

❧ If a steamy atmosphere isn't especially helpful, try opening a window to allow some fresh air into the room. In some cases this reduces swelling of the vocal chords, making it easier for your child to breathe.

❧ If the child is older than three, they may respond well to a warm vervain infusion (one teabag to one pot of hot water). Give one teaspoon of the warm, strained infusion as often as feels soothing, always checking the temperature on the back of your hand first.

CAUTION!

IF ANY OF THE FOLLOWING OCCUR, GET EMERGENCY MEDICAL ASSISTANCE:
- **Severe breathing difficulties accompanied by pale, clammy, blue-tinged skin around the face and lips**

TYPE OF CROUP	GENERAL SYMPTOMS	WORSE FROM	BETTER FOR	REMEDY NAME
Croup that develops or gets more intense after midnight	- Symptoms get noticeably worse when lying down - Cough triggers hoarseness, retching and possible vomiting - Child clutches his or her sides with the effort of coughing	- Talking - Bending forward - Cold drinks	- Firm pressure - Contact with fresh air	**Drosera**
Harsh cough that comes on after exposure to dry, cold winds	- Child seems fine during the day but wakes during the night in great anxiety and distress - Symptoms are aggravated by panic and restlessness - Breathing is made difficult by very dry, hoarse cough	- Contact with very cold winds or smoky atmospheres - Cold drinks - During the night (especially after midnight)	- Breaking into a sweat - Stable, moderate temperatures	**Aconite**
Croup with stringy mucus that only comes up with a great effort	- Lots of breathlessness, gagging and retching with distressing coughing spasms - When it eventually is raised, mucus looks yellow and sticky - Cold, damp weather aggravates symptoms.	- On waking - Bending forwards - Taking clothes off - Being chilled	- Moving about - Moderate warmth	**Kali bich**
Croup that is at its most intense on falling asleep	- Cough with croup that sounds rasping, dry and harsh - Breathing in is difficult when feeling agitated	- Sugary food or drink - Talking - Being touched - Inhaling - Cold drinks	- Sips of warm drinks	**Spongia**

ear infections

Children are more susceptible to ear infections and earache because the eustachian tube, which runs from the back of the nose to the ear, is proportionally shorter in children than in adults and, as a result, infection can be rapidly transferred from the nasal passages to the ears. Common symptoms of ear infections can include any combination of the following:

- **In babies and toddlers who can't use verbal communication to describe what's wrong, watch out for any pulling or rubbing at the ears**
- **Episodes of sharp, stabbing pain in the ear(s)**
- **Reduced hearing from a sense of fullness in the affected ear(s)**
- **If the condition results in a perforation of the eardrum, a discharge will trickle visibly from the affected ear**
- **A raised temperature, lethargy and a general sense of being listless and unwell**

Conventional treatment consists of a course of antibiotics to be taken either orally or in the form of ear drops. If any of the following measures are brought into play at the very first twinge of an ear problem, they should prevent the condition progressing further. However, if these strategies do not resolve the situation, they can be used as additional complementary support together with conventional treatment. If your child begins to show signs of repeated bouts of ear infections that require regular treatment with antibiotics, consider consulting a homeopath who should be able to eliminate the underlying weakness in your child's constitution that is leaving them vulnerable to re-infection.

practical self-help

❧ Apply a warm compress to sensitive, painful ears. Immerse a clean flannel in warm water. Wring it out well and hold it against the affected ear until it cools down.
❧ If you know your child is vulnerable to recurrent ear problems, always make sure they wear a hat or scarf in cold windy weather that covers the ears well.
❧ Prevent the affected ear or ears from getting wet.
❧ A few teaspoonfuls of chamomile tea can help calm toddlers and young children who feel fractious and restless with earache.

CAUTION!
Severe pain in the ear combined with a high temperature in an obviously poorly child should be promptly checked out by your doctor

TYPE OF EAR PROBLEM	GENERAL SYMPTOMS	WORSE FROM	BETTER FOR	REMEDY NAME
Earache that's set off by a difficult episode of teething	- Child is fractious with pain - Yells and screams and won't be distracted - One cheek looks pale while the other is flushed when feverish	- During the night - Becoming chilled or contact with cold draughts - Becoming overheated	- Being carried or rocked - Warmth locally applied to painful side - Being taken out for a short drive	**Chamomilla**
Earache that sets in shortly after exposure to dry, cold winds	- Child plays happily in the fresh air during the day but wakes during the night restless and panicky with ear pain - Feverish with hot head and cool body	- Contact with extreme cold or heat - Loud noise - Waking during the night	- Moderate temperatures - Sweating	**Aconite**
Rapidly developing high temperature with earache	- Skin feels hot and dry with fever and looks red and flushed - Ear pain may be worse on, or restricted to, the right side - Ear pain is associated with swollen glands and sore throat, which may also be worse on the right side	- Jarring movement - Too much excitement - Becoming chilled	- Resting in a quiet room - Warmth locally applied to the painful part	**Belladonna**
Early stage of earache with itchy feeling in the affected ear	- Although onset of ear pain is rapid, symptoms are less dramatic than those needing Aconite or Belladonna - Symptoms may be worse on, or restricted to, the left side	- Contact with cold draughts - During the night - Moving around - Being touched	- Cool compresses - Resting quietly	**Ferrum phos**
Earache that sets in as a stage of an established head cold	- Thick, yellowish-green mucus congestion with swollen glands - Sore throat with sharp, sticking pains on the same side as earache - Very sensitive to being chilled and comforted by warmth	- Becoming chilled - Uncovering the painful ear(s) - In the autumn and winter	- Humidity - Keeping the head warm in cold weather - Warmth applied to the painful part	**Hepar sulph**

snuffles

This rather imprecise term is used to describe general congestion in babies and young children that often follows a bad cold. The kind of mucus produced varies and can be clear and runny or thick and yellowish-green that has a tendency to dry around the edges of the nostrils in a rather nasty-looking crusty deposit. Children who suffer periodically from snuffles may also be inclined to mouth breathe and/or snore at night due to having a persistently blocked up nose.

Snuffles on their own will not usually require conventional medical treatment, but if your doctor diagnoses an additional bacterial infection in the ear, throat or chest they are likely to prescribe a course of antibiotics. Recurrent mucus congestion in older children may be treated with decongestant medication and any of the following may be used safely in combination with conventional medication. However, if you feel that you child is subject to perpetual snuffles that are undermining his or her health on an on-going basis, it is worth consulting a homeopathic practitioner who should be able to remove the underlying tendency to the problem.

practical self-help

❧ Echinacea is now available in a formula that's especially suited to children. This herbal preparation is excellent for supporting the immune system and can help your child fight any residual symptoms after a cold hasn't quite cleared up. Follow the directions for dosage on the product until the infection has cleared and resume as soon as another cold shows signs of developing.

❧ Cut down on dairy products and sugary foods that aggravate mucus congestion and substitute with vitamin C-rich fresh fruit and vegetables.

❧ If breathing is congested at night, humidify the atmosphere in the your child's bedroom by using a custom-made humidifier, or place a bowl of cold water near each radiator or heater.

❧ Congestion in the nose and chest can be eased by encouraging your child to sleep slightly propped up on two or three pillows.

❧ Vaporising a drop or two of peppermint, lemon or tea tree essential oils can help clear congestion.

CAUTION!

If snuffles are associated with noticeable congestion and wheezing in your child's chest that makes it difficult for them to breathe, consult your doctor

TYPE OF SNUFFLES	GENERAL SYMPTOMS	WORSE FROM	BETTER FOR	REMEDY NAME
Greenish-yellow mucus that causes distress in overheated surroundings	- Child is clingy, weepy and generally in need of lots of sympathy and attention when under the weather - Nasal congestion leads to a very dry mouth and yellowish-coated tongue	- Fatty foods - Stuffy rooms - Lying in bed at night - Being indoors	- Gentle exercise in the fresh air - Well ventilated rooms - Cold drinks	**Pulsatilla**
Snuffles with yellow-coloured mucus that's slightly blood-streaked	- Uncomfortable dry sensation inside the nostrils with persistent nasal obstruction - Nose looks red, shiny and feels sore to the touch - Symptoms get progressively worse as the evening comes on	- Becoming chilled - Lying on the left side - Getting overexcited	- Warmth - Massage - Attention and reassurance	**Phosphorus**
Snuffles with very stringy, difficult to move mucus	- Uncomfortable, blocked feeling in the nostrils with a persistent drip that runs down the back of the nose to the throat - Peculiar sensation of a hair irritating the back of the tongue	- Contact with damp - Becoming chilled - Stooping - Waking from sleep	- Warmth - Resting in bed - Firm pressure	**Kali bich**

homeopathy

bed-wetting

This problem can arise for a number of physical or psychological reasons that make it difficult for a child's nervous system to exert the necessary control over their bladder. Common reasons may include:

- **A low-grade bladder infection**
- **Mechanical triggers, such as kidney dysfunction**
- **High stress levels or feeling generally insecure or nervous**

Even if your child isn't completely dry at night by the age of three, bear in mind that roughly ten per cent of children are still damp at night by the age of five. As a general guide, if your child is showing no signs of having bladder control during the day or night by the time of their fourth birthday you may want to get a medical opinion.

Any of the following can help with a temporary relapse in bed-wetting when the child has been under a lot of stress. However, for longer term problems, it would be worthwhile to get a professional assessment.

practical self-help

❧ Where possible, and especially if the problem appears to be stress-related, avoid reacting in a way that is going to make your child feel tense or guilty as this will more than likely lead to it happening again. It is also a good idea to keep dry nightwear and fresh sheets close to hand so as to minimise feelings of frustration in the middle of the night.

❧ If with older children you suspect that stress is responsible, then it is worth considering counselling as long as your child feels comfortable about the idea of talking through issues.

❧ Mechanical devices, such as a pad or buzzer, can alert your child to the fact that they're having an accident and need to go to the loo. You can also use a star chart to help you and your child identify if there are any obvious patterns to the frequency and severity of the bedwetting.

❧ Controversy reigns over whether lifting a child during the night to take them to the toilet, or restricting their fluid intake before it's time for bed does any good at all.

CAUTION!

If your child is normally dry at night but begins to wet the bed while also complaining of stinging or pain on passing water, see your doctor who may want to test a urine sample for infection

TYPE OF BED-WETTING	GENERAL SYMPTOMS	WORSE FROM	BETTER FOR	REMEDY NAME
Bed-wetting that sets in after getting chilled and damp	- Lying on the back makes the urge to urinate almost impossible to resist - A leaky bladder can lead to dribbling of urine when coughing sneezing or laughing - Weepy and clingy when realises an accident has happened	- Lying flat on the back - Damp chill - Getting overheated at night	- Contact with fresh air - Well ventilated rooms	**Pulsatilla**
Bed-wetting in sensitive children after an emotional shock	- An escalation of stress in anxious, timid children who are inclined to be rigid or obsessive	- Becoming chilled - Emotional stress	- Being wrapped up warmly	**Silica**
Bed-wetting that occurs on falling asleep	- Child is emotionally sensitive and nervous with a fear of going to bed in the dark - Restless sleep with bad dreams - Physically restless at night with a tendency for the legs to be constantly on the go	- Contact with dry, cold winds - After getting soaked	- Warmth in general	**Causticum**

childhood infectious diseases

The debate about the most effective and safest management of childhood illnesses, such as measles, mumps and whooping cough is an extremely emotive one. The decision whether to vaccinate a child or not is very serious and should not be taken lightly. However, it is worth pointing out that homeopathic treatment can have a great deal to offer in supporting a child through a mild case of any of the common infectious diseases, whether they have been vaccinated or not.

Homeopathic remedies are understood to work by stimulating the body's own, self-healing mechanism and therefore they are an equally valid option of treatment for viral or bacterial infections. This is in sharp contrast to conventional medicine, which has a wide range of anti-bacterial medication at its disposal but few anti-virals. As infections such as measles and chicken pox are viral in origin, homeopathic support has a great deal to offer in supporting your child through each stage of these illnesses, which can give rise to symptoms of feverishness, general aches and pains and irritation of the skin. Perhaps most significantly of all, appropriate homeopathic prescribing can play a very practical role in speeding up recovery and potentially shortening the duration of illness.

the vaccination debate

The conventional medical position states that vaccination is an invaluable way of protecting babies and children from the possible side-effects of contagious children's illnesses such as mumps, measles or whooping cough. Although a very small percentage of children may be considered too high risk to vaccinate (such as those with a history of severe allergic reactions), immunisation is considered as generally being advisable for most children.

The alternative/complementary medical perspective presents a different viewpoint, suggesting that for some children there may be drawbacks associated with vaccination that are more subtle than the extreme neurological reactions that are considered to be a relatively rare occurrence. These more low-grade symptoms are thought to be linked to low immunity and include ear problems, recurrent infections and an aggravation of allergic skin conditions, such as eczema.

Problems are also thought to occur as a result of the different mechanisms involved when immunity is generated in response to vaccination, rather than acquired naturally. With the latter, infections usually enter the body via the mucus membranes of the nose and mouth before they begin to circulate in the bloodstream. For example, with measles a child will generally inhale the virus through the nose and it will spread and multiply through the tonsils, adenoids and lymph nodes before entering the bloodstream. As a consequence, the virus has made contact with the spleen, liver, thymus gland and bone marrow before symptoms begin to emerge and the immune system is stimulated to respond to the body as a whole.

Vaccines, however, are usually injected directly into the bloodstream, and many complementary practitioners consider that this has a very stressful effect on the immune system. Furthermore, babies and infants are regularly exposed to this process during the first year of life when the immune system is considered to be in the process of developing and, therefore, the possible negative effects do deserve consideration.

Ultimately the decision rests with the child's parents, and so it is essential that fair, balanced information is made available to use as a basis for discussion with your doctor or health visitor (see suggested reading on page 282). Above all else, it is important to remember that this is not a stark either/or situation as parents may choose to prepare their child with homeopathic treatment in advance of vaccination, and continue with homeopathic support if any symptoms, such as recurrent respiratory congestion, arise after treatment.

mumps

This is an extremely uncomfortable viral illness that starts with an incubation period of approximately two to four weeks. Initial symptoms can include any combination of the following:

- **A vague sense of being unwell and under the weather**
- **Feverishness**
- **Listlessness**

Later symptoms include:

- **Swollen, painful glands that are located under the ears**
- **Sensitive salivary glands under the jaw and the tongue**
- **Difficulty with swallowing and chewing**
- **Swelling and discomfort may affect both sides equally or be limited to one side of the face and neck**

It is important to ensure that children who are known to have mumps avoid contact with adults who have never had the illness as in men it can trigger extremely painful testicular swelling and in women it can cause inflammation of the ovaries, which interferes with fertility.

practical self-help

❧ Apply a warm compress to swollen, tender glands in the face or neck. Wrap a hot water bottle in a soft cloth or thin towel or wring out a warm, wet flannel and hold it to the sensitive area.

❧ Spritz the warm compress with lavender hydrosol water for a soothing and comforting effect.

❧ Make sure that your child drinks enough fluid in order to keep their temperature down as much as possible. Avoid acidic, citrus drinks that make the salivary glands work hard and, to reduce the discomfort of opening the mouth too wide, provide a straw and purée any foods first in a blender.

CAUTION!
IF ANY OF THE FOLLOWING OCCUR, GET EMERGENCY MEDICAL ASSISTANCE:
- **Stiffness of the neck accompanied by a very severe headache and/or convulsions**
- **Vomiting that is accompanied by pains in the abdomen**

Homeopathic Support Table overleaf

TYPE OF MUMPS	GENERAL SYMPTOMS	WORSE FROM	BETTER FOR	REMEDY NAME
Swift onset of symptoms that are noticeably more severe on the right side	- Very high temperature with flushed, dry skin that radiates heat - Throat is painful which makes swallowing difficult - Normally placid child becomes unusually irritable and bad-tempered	- Stooping - Bright light - Jarring movement - Becoming chilled	- Resting propped up in bed - Peace and quiet - Moderate warmth	**Belladonna**
Slow, insidious onset of symptoms over several days	- Marked thirst with low-grade dehydration leads to dry skin, mouth and lips - Associated headache and constipation - A tendency for everything to feel much worse for even the slightest movement	- Becoming overheated - Moving - Making physical effort of any kind	- Resting in one position - Sweating - Long, cold drinks - Being kept comfortably cool	**Bryonia**
Established stage of mumps with severe stiffness and inflammation of the glands	- Severe tenderness and sensitivity of the glands in front of the ears makes moving the jaw excruciatingly painful - As a result, talking, eating and drinking cause great distress - Irritating dry sensation at the back of the throat with marked thirst	- On the left side - Sweating - Becoming too cold		**Jaborandi**
Tight, stiff feeling under the ears and jaw	- The tonsils and uvula at the back of the throat look puffy and inflamed - Swallowing is very painful as a result of persistent dryness in the throat	- Severe chill - At night - Becoming overheated	- Moderate temperatures	**Phytolacca**
Lingering symptoms at the end of the illness	- This remedy can be very helpful once the feverish stage has passed	- Sweating - At night - Extremes of warmth or cold	- Consistent moderate temperatures	**Mercurius**

chicken pox

This viral infection is preceded by quite a long incubation period (one to three weeks) before the characteristic symptoms appear. However, once they make an appearance, the signs are very distinctive and can include any of the following:

- **Flu-type symptoms, with listlessness, shivering, and general vague aches and pains**
- **A rash that looks raised and blistery; as though water were trapped under each spot**
- **Spots are likely to make their first appearance on the trunk, spreading rapidly to the back, arms, head, face and legs**
- **With a severe bout, spots that are very itchy on the surface of the skin can also internally affect the throat, genitals and ears, feeling sensitive and painful rather than itchy**
- **At the last stage the spots dry out and become more crusty as they get less itchy**

practical self-help

❧ During the phase when your child has flu-type symptoms, keep their fluid intake up and don't worry too much if they are not hungry at this stage.

❧ Don't encourage your child to soak in a hot bath when the spots are in the process of emerging as this can lead to an unpleasant sense of enervation and exhaustion. Instead, sponge your child down as frequently as they want in a room that's comfortably warm.

❧ Swabbing with a diluted tincture of Calendula (one part tincture to ten parts boiled, cooled water) soothes itchy spots while also discouraging infection from setting in to any that have lost their tops through towel drying or scratching.

❧ After swabbing with the tincture, apply Calendula cream to extend the soothing effect.

❧ Once bathing feels comfortable, soak in an oatmeal bath. Place a generous handful of oats in a small bag of muslin or gauze and run the warm water through as the bath fills.

❧ Avoid giving aspirin to your child as a way of reducing a high temperature as it can lead to a condition called Reye's syndrome which involves drowsiness, feverishness, vomiting, loss of consciousness and convulsions and appears to be linked to children under twelve years of age taking aspirin.

CAUTION!

IF ANY OF THE FOLLOWING OCCUR, GET EMERGENCY MEDICAL ASSISTANCE:

- **Extreme lethargy or weakness combined with rapid, laboured or shallow breathing**
- **Convulsions or vomiting**
- **Any signs of bleeding beneath the skin**
- **A persistent and/or severe headache especially if combined with a stiff neck**

TYPE OF CHICKEN POX	GENERAL SYMPTOMS	WORSE FROM	BETTER FOR	REMEDY NAME
Rapid onset of fever with marked restlessness and anxiety. Usually needed before there is any sign of the rash	- Thirsty and dry-skinned with high temperature - Finds discomfort of being unwell intolerable - Normally placid child becomes panicky and fearful	- At night - Moving from extremely warm to cold environment	- Sweating - Sound rest - Fresh air that doesn't chill	**Aconite**
Rapidly developing high temperature with flushed, bright red skin	- This is well indicated before the rash emerges but when the feverishness is more dramatic than that requiring Aconite - Skin looks bright red, feels dry and radiates heat - Marked irritability and grouchiness	- Becoming chilled - Being disturbed - Jarring movement - Loud noise - Bright light	- Resting by lying propped up in bed - Peace and quiet - Subdued lighting	**Belladonna**
Slow-to-develop rash with severe or lingering cough	- Spots are slow to emerge and are large and tinged bluish-purple - Also slow to clear and leave a red mark - Coated tongue with rattling chesty cough	- Warm bathing - Becoming overheated - Heat in general - Lying down	- Bringing up phlegm - Keeping comfortably cool	**Ant tart**
Unbearably itchy spots at night that make sleep impossible	- Restless at night with constant tossing and turning in bed in effort to get comfortable - Indicated for spots that become moist or crusty and are aggravated by contact with cold, damp air	- After scratching - In bed at night - Keeping still - Undressing	- Warm, dry conditions - Rubbing - Changing position	**Rhus tox**
Established stage of illness with lingering rash	- Although chilly, reacts very badly to stuffy, overheated environments - Dry mouth without thirst but with a white-coated tongue - Contented, easygoing child becomes clingy and weepy	- When resting - Later in the day and evening - Stuffy, overheated rooms	- Cool bathing - Applying a cool compress - Cold food and drink - Having lots of cuddles	**Pulsatilla**

measles

This is a very infectious viral illness that will incubate for roughly ten days to two weeks. Like chicken pox, it begins with fairly general symptoms of being off-colour, listless and feverish with maybe a dry cough, sensitive eyes and a runny nose. However, once passed the initial stage, the following symptoms are likely to develop:

- **Small ulcer-like eruptions inside the mouth that look a little like grains of salt**
- **Continuing feverishness**
- **A raised, red rash that appears initially behind the ears before moving down over the trunk**
- **As the spots cover the body, they increase in size**
- **Once the spots have come out fully, the temperature should come down**

Conventional medicine advocates vaccination as a way of preventing the onset of a dose of measles, rather than having any specific anti-viral medication at its disposal. If your child has caught the disease, even when they have been immunised against it, the following self-help advice can be extremely valuable.

practical self-help

- Make sure your child drinks lots of fluid as dehydration will only make the fever worse.
- If your child has a nasty cough, avoid milky drinks that can aggravate mucus congestion.
- Once appetite returns, introduce light, digestible foods again.
- If eyes feel sore and sensitive, soak two cotton wool pads in cool water before squeezing them almost dry and resting them on closed eyes until they warm up.
- Calamine lotion is an effective temporary soothant to itchy skin although it also tends to dry the skin out. Try swabbing irritated spots with cotton wool pads soaked in Calendula tincture (one part tincture to ten parts boiled, cooled water) instead.
- Once spots feels soothed by the diluted tincture, apply Calendula cream to maintain the soothing effect on the skin.

CAUTION!
IF ANY OF THE FOLLOWING OCCUR, GET EMERGENCY MEDICAL ASSISTANCE:

- **Marked sensitivity to light**
- **Vomiting with stiff neck and/or persistent headache**
- **Bleeding from any orifice or under the skin**
- **Severe pains in the ears**
- **Severe coughing with difficulty breathing**
- **A high temperature remaining after the rash has fully emerged, or if you feel your child isn't visibly improving by this stage and showing signs of weakness or severe, persistent lethargy**

Homeopathic Support Table overleaf

TYPE OF MEASLES	GENERAL SYMPTOMS	WORSE FROM	BETTER FOR	REMEDY NAME
Sudden emergence of symptoms during the night	- This remedy is most useful in the first, feverish stage of infection - Sensitive eyes with harsh, croupy cough and clear running nose - Fever peaks speedily with lots panicky restlessness	- During the night - Extreme change of temperature	- Sound sleep - Contact with comfortably cool air that doesn't chill	**Aconite**
First stage of illness with very high temperature	- Skin is flushed, bright red, dry and radiates heat - Rapid pulse with fast-developing temperature - Ordinarily placid, happy child becomes irritable and peevish	- Noise - Being disturbed - Bright light - Jarring - Becoming chilled	- Subdued lighting - Comfortable levels of warmth - Peace and quiet	**Belladonna**
Second stage of measles with very sensitive eyes	- Very sensitive, burning, watery eyes - Nose runs in sympathy but nasal discharge is bland in comparison to the tears - Both eye and nasal irritation respond favourably to contact with cool, fresh air	- Warmth - In the evenings - Exposure to bright light	- Cool, fresh air - Wiping the eyes	**Euphrasia**
Slow, insidious development of symptoms with dry, irritating cough	- High temperature develops slowly - Severe headache responds badly to even the slightest movement - Low-grade dehydration leads to dry mouth, dry skin and constipation - Child becomes withdrawn, prostrated and irritable	- Eating - Becoming hot - Movement	- Keeping in one position - Long, cold drinks - Firm pressure to painful areas	**Bryonia**
Last stage of measles with thick, yellowy-green congestion	- Rash has fully come out and the temperature has gone down - Mouth feels dry and coated but with no thirst as a result - Contented child becomes unusually demanding, weepy and clingy	- Getting overheated - Warm drinks - Lying in bed - Approach of evening or night	- Contact with fresh air - Cool compresses - Gentle movement - Hugs and affection	**Pulsatilla**

whooping cough

This is a highly contagious viral illness that has an incubation period of approximately one week to a fortnight. Initial symptoms may include a slight cough, a high temperature, nasal discharge and a feeling of lethargy. However, by the second stage of the illness the following symptoms will emerge:

- **Thick nasal discharge**
- **A characteristic cough that ends in a whooping sound and a sensation of breathlessness**
- **Vomiting, often at the end of an especially nasty attack of coughing**
- **Flushing and discolouration of the face from the sheer effort of coughing**
- **The tendency to cough may last for anything up to six months after the initial infection**

Conventional medicine recommends immunisation, rather than having a range of treatments on offer to reduce the distress of symptoms should they arise. Complementary medical practitioners can do a great deal to support a child through a bout of whooping cough but this treatment needs to be administered by an experienced practitioner to ensure success.

practical self-help

❧ The distress of severe episodes of coughing can be very alarming to a young child and speaking in a soothing, calming voice can do a great deal to ease the panic and get the coughing bout over more quickly.

❧ If vomiting seems to happen as a result of a severe coughing bout, give your child something small to eat after a major attack as this gives it the best chance of staying down.

❧ Cough-suppressant medicines should be avoided as they congest the lungs with mucus. However unpleasant the coughing is, it is essential for expelling mucus from the lungs that would otherwise aggravate symptoms of breathlessness.

❧ Food and drink made with cow's milk should be avoided as it aggravates mucus congestion, while also being hard to digest. Also give sugary food and drink a wide berth.

❧ If your child isn't keen to eat because of the distress of recurrent bouts of vomiting, soothe the stomach with a few sips of grape juice which is good for the digestion.

CAUTION!

IF ANY OF THE FOLLOWING OCCUR, GET EMERGENCY MEDICAL ASSISTANCE:

- **Whooping cough in a baby younger than six months**
- **Episodes of wheezing, accelerated and/or laboured breathing**
- **Marked drowsiness and/or lethargy combined with a severe headache**

Homeopathic Support Table overleaf

TYPE OF WHOOPING COUGH	GENERAL SYMPTOMS	WORSE FROM	BETTER FOR	REMEDY NAME
Episodes of coughing that start at bedtime	- Child is cold and clammy and vomits during bouts of coughing - Coughing begins with sense of irritation and tickling in the throat - Choking sensation with cough	- Resting on a pillow - Second half of the night - Cold food - Laughing	- Fresh air - Firm pressure	**Drosera**
Whooping cough with spasmodic bouts of coughing ending in vomiting of stringy mucus	- Nasty sensation of smothering sets in before a severe coughing bout; often triggered by the process of eating - Difficulty in finding a comfortable, stable temperature: feels too hot when covered, too chilly when covers are taken off	- Breathing in - Eating - Feeling too hot or too cold	- Moderate temperatures	**Corallium rubrum**
Whooping cough with severe congestion in the chest that leads to a rattling cough	- Big effort needed to raise mucus during a coughing spasm - Child bends backwards in an effort to raise phlegm - Feels more comfortable sitting up since this allows mucus to drain more effectively	- Milk - Lying down - Movement - Getting angry and irritable	- Sitting up - Raising mucus - Burping - After vomiting	**Ant tart**
Whooping cough with coughing bouts triggered by overly warm rooms	- Child's face becomes dusky, purple-red in colour as a result of severe coughing spasms - Constant swallowing in an effort to try and clear the throat of congestion and mucus - When mucus does come up it looks clear and sticky	- Touch or pressure to the throat - Irritation of the throat - Brushing teeth - Overheated rooms	- Walking - Cold drinks - Coolness locally applied	**Coccus cacti**
Whooping cough with severe coughing that leads to complete exhaustion	- Coughing quickly turns from harsh and dry to loose and mucusy - Due to the effort of coughing, child looks pale, exhausted and sweaty and feels clammy	- Heat - When speaking - Lack of ventilation - Heavy clothes	- Being fanned - Loosening clothes - After sleep	**Carbo veg**

school phobia

This can be a particular problem in September with the beginning of the school year, especially when children are making the transition from one school to another or contemplating a stressful academic year ahead with important and difficult exams. Children who are most likely to be affected are those who struggle with the prospect of change and take some time to adjust to new situations and challenges. Symptoms will vary from one child to another but any of the following can be interpreted as signs of distress:

- **Poor sleep quality or problems in initially getting to sleep**
- **Mood swings, including uncharacteristic reserve, weepiness or irritability**
- **Problems with concentration and mental focus**
- **Digestive upsets including nausea and/or diarrhoea, or a sensation of butterflies in the stomach**

There's a good chance that for most children this will just be a phase that will end by itself once they have adjusted to the change. However, appropriate homeopathic prescribing can do a great deal to speed up this natural process, making the whole experience far less distressing for the child and their family. As always, problems that are very severe or well established will call for professional homeopathic support rather than home prescribing.

practical self-help

❧ Avoid fizzy colas, sweets and chocolate biscuits that can aggravate mood swings. Substitute with healthy, energy-balancing alternatives such as fresh vegetables, fruit juices, smoothies, unroasted nuts and seeds.

❧ For older children, try giving soothing herbal tea blends, such as chamomile, valerian, and passiflora, as preparation for a sound night's sleep.

❧ Add a few drops of clary sage, geranium, ylang ylang or lavender essential oil to a warm bath as a gentle way of unwinding after a stressful day at school. Alternatively vaporise a sparing number of drops in a custom-made oil burner in your child's room.

CAUTION!

IF ANY OF THE FOLLOWING OCCUR, CONSULT YOUR DOCTOR:

- **Persistent low moods that show no sign of lifting or only get worse and more disruptive**
- **Any suggestion on your child's part that they are being bullied**
- **Lack of appetite on a long term basis**
- **Difficulty in going to sleep or achieving a refreshing deep sleep**

Homeopathic Support Table overleaf

TYPE OF SCHOOL PHOBIA	GENERAL SYMPTOMS	WORSE FROM	BETTER FOR	REMEDY NAME
Agitated anxiety with fidgets and a constant need to chat	- Severe restlessness with palpitations and trembling - Cravings for sweet things as a comfort when anxiety levels are high only aggravate symptoms, in particular stomach upsets and nervous diarrhoea	- On waking - Hot stuffy rooms - In the night - Thinking about going back to school	- Contact with fresh air - Belching	**Argentum nitricum**
Intense anxiety on the verge of a panic attack	- Anxiety symptoms descend very rapidly and pass away as quickly - Fear is either linked to a very specific aspect of returning to school, or is very general - Emotional, restless and fearful during the night	- Emotional shock - Loud, disruptive noise - Becoming overheated or chilled	- Moderate temperatures	**Aconite**
Anticipatory anxiety with painless diarrhoea	- Uptight and withdrawn with anxiety and lack of confidence - Weak and chilly with diarrhoea	- Brooding on stressful events - Becoming overheated - Physical exertion	- Rest - Distraction	**Gelsemium**
Extreme restlessness, queasiness and cramping diarrhoea	- Very upset when routine and sense of order is threatened - Anxiety symptoms are especially severe at night and in the early hours of the morning - Well indicated for children who are competitive, neat and perfectionist when under stress	- Darkness - When alone - Untidy surroundings - Becoming chilled	- Fresh air to the head and face while the body is warm - Warmth - Sips of a warm drink	**Arsenicum album**
Problems falling asleep due to anxiety about school work	- Recurrent tension headaches and/or constipation - Finds it difficult to mentally switch off although feeling overtired	- Getting too hot - Physical effort and exertion - Feeling under stress and pressure	- Cooling off - Long, cold drinks - Peace and quiet - Warmth	**Bryonia**

TYPE OF SCHOOL PHOBIA	GENERAL SYMPTOMS	WORSE FROM	BETTER FOR	REMEDY NAME
Irritable and short-fused when under pressure	- Once asleep, dreams about worries and focus of stress - Sleeps fitfully until it's time to wake, when drifts into the soundest sleep - Feels groggy on waking - This remedy can help break the negative cycle for children who work late and can't sleep soundly as a result	- When it's time to get up - Noisy disruptive surroundings - Caffeinated drinks	- Peace and quiet	**Nux vomica**
Weepiness and clinginess in shy, bashful children	- Emotional at the prospect of getting used to a new school term - Moods change quickly from tears to laughter depending on the amount of sympathetic company around - Headaches and digestive upsets are common stress-induced reactions	- Overheated, stuffy rooms - Feeling lonely and neglected - When left alone to think	- Having a good cry - Sympathy and attention - Taking a gentle walk in the fresh air	**Pulsatilla**

homeopathy

225

german measles

Also known as rubella, this is generally quite a mild illness that involves a feeling of being under the weather combined with a slight rash. In addition, any of the following symptoms are a possibility:

- **Feverishness**
- **A flatish, small, pinky rash that often appears first on the face, spreading quickly to the rest of the body**
- **Swollen glands at the base of the neck and/or behind the ears**

For advice on complementary and homeopathic strategies for dealing with German measles, see the information given in the 'Measles' section.

CAUTION!

Although this illness is extremely mild in comparison with other infectious illnesses, it must be stressed that there is a specific danger in relation to this disease as German measles has been connected with possible birth defects in the unborn foetus. Therefore it is very important that any child known to be suffering with this illness has no contact with a pregnant woman for the duration of the illness. For this reason, always inform any family members, friends and colleagues if you suspect your child is incubating, or has actually developed, German measles.

IF ANY OF THE FOLLOWING OCCUR, GET EMERGENCY MEDICAL ASSISTANCE:
- **A long-lasting headache, especially if combined with a stiff neck and vomiting**
- **Breathing difficulties**
- **Extreme distress or malaise**

1 | homeopathy and emotional healing

Positive emotional health is a guiding principle of homeopathic treatment and therefore, irrespective of the physical problem that may have brought you to the consulting room, a homeopath will always spend time during your appointment assessing the quality of your emotional and mental health.

From a homeopathic perspective, positive health is enjoyed when an equilibrium between the mind and body is achieved and maintained. In this state, you have physical energy and vitality and feel that everyday challenges can be tackled readily, with enthusiasm and without the stress that overwhelms you when you are feeling run down.

High, poorly managed stress levels are often responsible for escalating emotional problems and therefore a significant proportion of this chapter looks at effective ways to prevent and/or cope with stress-related emotional illness. As with the other conditions dealt with in this book, the emotional symptoms that are treated most successfully by the home prescriber are those that fall into an 'acute' category. In other words, they are of recent onset and can be traced to a specific triggering factor rather than being an entrenched aspect of the personality or constitution.

The latter generally fall into a longer term category of illness that can be classed as 'chronic'. This kind of emotional illness can be very debilitating and, in some cases, have serious consequences when not treated appropriately. Therefore chronic emotional illnesses are best dealt with by an experienced homeopathic practitioner while mild to moderate emotional conditions of recent onset should be greatly eased by a combination of acute homeopathic prescribing and the following complementary self-help measures.

anticipatory anxiety

Anticipatory anxiety is common when a stressful event is looming on the horizon. This can include anything that puts you under extra pressure, such as giving a last-minute presentation at work or going on an important first date. Symptoms can include any of the following and may occur in any combination and with varying levels of intensity:

- **Palpitations (awareness of fluttering or rapid heartbeat)**
- **Difficulties with mentally switching off and relaxing**
- **Sleep disturbance**
- **Lack of appetite or strong food cravings**
- **Nausea**
- **Diarrhoea or loose stools**
- **Inability to mentally focus and concentrate**
- **Easy perspiration**
- **Irritability when under pressure**

Any of the following are an excellent first port of call if you suffer when faced with a stressful event as these non-addictive strategies can provide a gentle but effective sense of calm, helping you to become more mentally focused and physically relaxed as a result.

practical self-help

❧ Learn how to breathe correctly. When pressure builds, without consciously knowing it, you are likely to take rapid, shallow breaths using only the upper part of your chest. As a result, the blood gases oxygen and carbon dioxide become imbalanced and feelings of tension and panic increase. Consciously relax your face, neck and shoulders as this allows the muscles of your chest to take in a deep lungful of air. Don't force the breath if you feel at all light headed or dizzy but simply get used to how it feels to breathe all the way from the lower part of your lungs to the top and rebalance your blood gases.

❧ Substitute alcohol, caffeine in any form and sugary food and drinks with calm-inducing herbal teas and always go for foods that have a high sedative content such as bananas, peanut butter, wholegrain cereals and breads and lettuce. Eat a small snack every couple of hours in order to keep blood sugar levels as stable as possible.

❧ Vaporise a few drops of calming essential oil, such as bergamot, chamomile, ylang ylang, clary sage, frankincense, and/or lavender in an aromatherapy burner.

❧ Rescue Remedy is a great, immediate restorative in the face of rising anxiety. Made from a blend of trauma-reducing flower essences, it can be sprayed directly onto the tongue, or diluted in a small glass of water and sipped as often as necessary.

TYPE OF ANXIETY	GENERAL SYMPTOMS	WORSE FROM	BETTER FOR	REMEDY NAME
Slow building anxiety with a tendency to feel withdrawn and unusually quiet	- Normally outgoing, chatty people become preoccupied when anxious - Symptoms build slowly and progressively as the day of the event gets nearer - Uneasy stomach with diarrhoea - Chilly, weak and shaky.	- Brooding - Overly warm surroundings	- Being effectively distracted - Cool, fresh air	**Gelsemium**
Rapid onset of major panic	- Panic symptoms come on quickly and severely - Thinking about the stressful situation causes such panic that fear of dying is a real problem - All symptoms are at their worst during the night, leading to very restless and disturbed sleep	- Building stress and pressure - Being too hot or too cold - Too much excitement - Waking from sleep at night	- Sound rest - Peace and quiet - Contact with fresh air	**Aconite**
Feeling anxious leads to an inability to stop talking	- Palpitations with trembling and feeling shaky all over - Craving for sugary foods that comfort in the short term, but make symptoms worse in the long run - Restlessness with upset stomach and diarrhoea	- Thinking about source of anxiety - During the night - Badly ventilated, stuffy rooms	- Contact with fresh air	**Arg nit**
'Free-floating' state of anxiety that attaches itself to any worry that's going around	- Normally extrovert, lively people become apathetic and drained of energy when over-anxious - Attention and affection from others help reduce distress of anxiety - Very sensitive to the feelings of others; can pick anxiety up from them	- Excessive excitement - In the early evening - Onset of darkness - Changes in atmospheric pressure	- Massage - Comfort - Reassurance - Soothing, calming company - Sound sleep	**Phosphorus**

homeopathy

●

229

Homeopathic Support Table continued overleaf

TYPE OF ANXIETY	GENERAL SYMPTOMS	WORSE FROM	BETTER FOR	REMEDY NAME
Anxiety as a result of living in the fast lane for too long	- Stressed out and anxious with an inability to relax, even at night - Aggravated by reliance on caffeine, cigarettes and/or alcohol in order to keep up the pace - Palpitations, poor sleep pattern and an emotional short fuse	- Stimulants - First thing in the morning - Becoming chilled - Too much noise - Feeling constipated	- Sound sleep - As the day goes on - Peace and quiet	**Nux vomica**
Anticipatory anxiety but with the ability to look calm and composed on the surface	- Anxious specifically about speaking in public; although terribly affected by nerves beforehand, the task, once under way, is likely to go very smoothly - Rumbling, gurgling and bloating in the belly and acidity and indigestion in the stomach	- In the middle of the afternoon - Thinking about the coming challenge - Lack of exercise	- Being distracted - Being comfortably warm without getting overheated	**Lycopodium**

CAUTION!

IF ANY OF THE FOLLOWING OCCUR, CONSULT YOUR DOCTOR:

• Anxiety symptoms that begin to seriously interfere with quality of life. This could involve severe sleep disturbance, erratic mood swings or lack of interest in socialising

• Symptoms of anxiety that develop without any obvious trigger

mild to moderate depression

It can be quite tricky to establish just what is meant by the word depression, as it is used to cover a wide spectrum of feelings that can vary considerably in severity and intensity. At the mildest end, it can describe a bout of the 'blues' that descends quickly, often in response to an upsetting trigger, and lifts as quickly as it came. At the sharp, most extreme end, it can equally well denote an episode of clinical depression that disrupts life and makes every day a genuine uphill struggle with negativity and distress.

Mild to moderate depression can be dealt with very effectively by using some of the practical strategies listed overleaf. More severe depression can also benefit from complementary medical approaches and yet these should be administered by a trained professional for they will be able to judge how the complementary support can work in conjunction with the conventional treatment that has been prescribed.

Symptoms of mild to moderate depression can vary greatly and may include any combination of the following:

- **Poor sleep quality and pattern**
- **Waking in the early hours of the morning**
- **Low physical, mental and emotional energy levels**
- **Reduced mental focus and concentration**
- **Lack of appetite or comfort eating**
- **Tearfulness or an inability to cry**
- **Feeling emotionally flat and unmotivated**
- **Mood swings including irritability, impatience and/or despondency**

Conventional medicine treats recurrent and/or severe bouts of depression with antidepressant drugs, perhaps combined with some kind of psychological therapy. Although many people are wary of antidepressants because of the negative press that has surrounded some of the newer SSRI formulas, it is worth stressing that, for very severe cases, these drugs provide essential mental and emotional breathing space. As a result of this respite, it can become possible to take the steps that are needed to improve quality of life. Although some forms of complementary medical support, and especially homeopathy, can be used very safely with any conventional prescriptions, take care with herbal medicines. Some herbal extracts, and in particular St John's Wort, does not interact positively in every case and I have included more advice on this issue in the section on St John's Wort overleaf.

practical self-help

❧ If a bout of the blues has descended, avoid foods and drinks that have a reputation for destabalising or lowering moods further. These include alcohol, coffee and anything with a very high white sugar content. Eat a small snack every couple of hours in order to balance blood sugar levels and have plenty of unrefined carbohydrates and fresh fruit and vegetables as these are good for lifting moods: salad greens, bananas, oranges, brown rice cakes and wholegrain brown bread are particularly beneficial.

❧ Although it will probably be the last thing you feel like doing, regular, rhythmic exercise is one of the most effective things you can do to boost a flagging mood as it stimulates the production of endorphins, the natural antidepressant chemicals in the body that also have pain-relieving properties. Choose from cycling, running, swimming, power walking or dancing and aim for five thirty-five-minute sessions a week.

❧ Although it's tempting to hide away when you are feeling low, stimulating, sensitive company can actually do you the world of good while being alone often gives you far too much time to brood on negative emotions.

❧ St John's Wort is a herbal supplement that has performed well in clinical trials for the treatment of mild to moderate depression. However, recent information has also suggested that this supplement may interfere with a small group of conventional drugs and therefore you should always consult your pharmacist or family doctor before self-medicating with this herbal extract. If you have had more than one episode of moderate depression but are not on any prescription drugs, it is still worth consulting a complementary practitioner before taking St. John's Wort.

❧ Specific essential aromatherapy oils have a mood-balancing effect and can provide very pleasurable emotional support when you are feeling down or fragile. Ylang ylang, clary sage, lavender, marjoram and/or chamomile can be added sparingly to a bath, used in a massage blend or vaporised to create an uplifting atmosphere.

CAUTION!

IF ANY OF THE FOLLOWING OCCUR, CONSULT YOUR DOCTOR:

- A phase of depression that refuses to lift or becomes steadily more intense
- Feelings of panic arising in connection with issues that would previously not have caused a problem when feeling yourself
- Noticeable apathy, indifference and lack of motivation that don't respond to positive stimuli
- Renewed feelings of strong depression in anyone who has suffered from the problem in the past
- Emotional numbness, isolation, or a feeling of unreality and disorientation
- Any suggestion that self-harm may be a possibility

TYPE OF DEPRESSION	GENERAL SYMPTOMS	WORSE FROM	BETTER FOR	REMEDY NAME
Withdrawn, inward feelings that follow an emotional loss	- This remedy can be immensely helpful for anyone who reacts with a 'stiff upper lip' to emotional stress - Emotions that are suppressed also reduce immune system functioning so cold sores or allergic symptoms can break out when feeling low	- Attention - Fuss - Sympathy - After crying (especially in public)	- Being alone - Cool surroundings - Fasting - Gentle exercise	**Natrum mur**
Bouts of the blues with temporary loss of libido	- Flatness and exhaustion - Feeling blue alternates with feeling strung out and unable to cope with daily demands	- After pregnancy - Approaching or during menopause - Making love - Emotional demands	- Aerobic exercise - Resting in a warm bed - Eating regularly to keep blood sugar levels stable	**Sepia**
Weepy and vulnerable when feeling blue	- This is the opposite picture to Natrum mur, as lots of physical affection and sympathy really has a positive effect when this remedy is needed - Mood quickly shifts from feeling low to cheerful in response to affection and emotional support	- Feeling neglected - In the evening and/or at night - Before a period or during pregnancy - Resting	- After having a good cry - Gentle exercise in the fresh air - Cooling off when feeling hemmed in and overheated	**Pulsatilla**
Bouts of the blues that arise from anger being suppressed	- Feeling emotionally low follows an upsetting event where feelings of anger have not been expressed - As a result, trivial things trigger an unjustified explosive outburst or hypersensitivity to criticism	- In the early hours of the morning - Slight touch - Making love	- Having a sound sleep - Warmth - Resting - After eating breakfast	**Staphysagria**

homeopathy

233

burn out

This is increasingly a pitfall of living in the twenty-first century. Pressures at work, especially when combined with a hectic social life, can usually be tolerated for a short period of time, although problems set in when this lifestyle becomes habitual. It is also worth noting that stress isn't always linked to the more negative pressures in life, like financial worries, or a tight deadline at work as being extremely busy and socially in demand can also be a strain. Stressful events also include the exciting changes in life, such as falling in love, moving house or getting that job you've always dreamed of, and these can catch anyone out because they are ultimately so positive.

The best way of combating burn out is to listen to what your body is telling you and to respond promptly when you feel you need to cut yourself some slack. If any combination of the following symptoms are becoming noticeable features of life, it's time to take action:

- **Mood swings**
- **Being on constant or persistent emotional short fuse**
- **Anxiety without any obvious trigger**
- **Feeling withdrawn**
- **General fatigue and lack of enthusiasm**
- **Recurrent minor infections**
- **General aches and pains**
- **Raised pulse rate**
- **A sense of being constantly on edge**

Conventional medicines can be used to treat some of these symptoms individually (e.g. anxiety). However, the risk with this approach is that the symptoms are only temporarily suppressed and the root cause remains, meaning that complications almost inevitably crop up further down the line.

The complementary medical approach is especially well suited to providing excellent support and if the problem is mild and of recent onset (within the last month or so), any of the following self-help measures will be of immense value. However, for more established and/or severe problems it is best to consult a trained complementary practitioner.

practical self-help

✺ As soon as you see the first signs and symptoms of burn out, review your daily work patterns to assess if you are over-challenged. If this is the case, take steps to manage your time more effectively by cutting back and delegating any inessential tasks and not saying an automatic 'yes' to everything. Take a lunch break rather than eating a sandwich at your desk. Leave the office and take a short walk or have a chat with colleagues about anything other than work. If you adopt these habits you will be surprised how more focused and productive you become when actually concentrating on your work.

❧ Take time every day to go through a guided relaxation exercise or learn how to meditate as both will help your mind and body relax so that you feel much more resilient when faced with a challenge.

❧ Regular exercise plays a very important part in balancing energy levels. Aim for three or four thirty-minute sessions a week rather than exhausting yourself in one epic two-hour session. Also make sure that you include a system of movement that is good for reducing stress symptoms, such as Tai chi, yoga, Pilates and power walking.

❧ Wild oats (Avena sativa), ginseng or vervain are all good herbal supplements for restoring flagging energy levels and may be taken as a diluted tincture, capsule or infusion. Wild oats are especially suitable during an extended period of high stress or a viral illness that's hit the system very hard.

❧ Always avoid relying on caffeine, nicotine, alcohol and junk food as a way of getting through a stressful day as these 'uppers' and 'downers' will only make matters worse in the long run. Their addictive, stimulant and mood-altering nature can magnify the symptoms of poor sleep, jitteriness, emotional-short fuse, lack of concentration and fatigue. Instead, support your immune system with good nutrition by
– eating as much antioxidant-rich fresh fruit and vegetables as you can manage
– eating regular portions of unrefined carbohydrates in the form of wholewheat cereals and brown rice
– eating small quantities of protein in the form of fresh fish and poultry and unroasted, unsalted nuts and seeds
– drinking green, herbal blends, fruit teas and plenty of filtered or still mineral water

CAUTION!

IF ANY OF THE FOLLOWING OCCUR, CONSULT YOUR DOCTOR OR:

• Growing introversion and withdrawal
• Preoccupation with control, such as radical weight loss and/or exercise regimes as a way of holding things together
• Inability to recover after a minor infectious illness or a tendency to recurrent infections
• Feeling low, depressed, negative and unable to cope with daily demands

Homeopathic Support Table overleaf

TYPE OF BURN OUT	GENERAL SYMPTOMS	WORSE FROM	BETTER FOR	REMEDY NAME
Physical exhaustion combined with marked digestive problems	- Often follows a very stressful event - Anxiety triggers bloating and gurgling with acid washing into the throat from the stomach - Becomes tense, hypercritical and domineering when afraid of failure	- Mental strain - Becoming too hot or cold - Tight clothing - From early afternoon to the early evening	- Gentle exercise - Sips of a warm drink - Being distracted from thinking about stressful stimuli	**Lycopodium**
Burn out with marked anxiety and restlessness at night with disturbed sleep pattern	- This remedy is valuable for anyone with a perfectionist streak - Falling short of high standards triggers anxiety when vulnerability, fears and phobias can escalate to the point of obsession - Compulsively neat and tidy about surroundings	- During the night - Cold in any form - Physical exertion - Alcohol	- Sitting propped up in bed in a freshly aired room - Company - Sips of a warm drink	**Arsenicum album**
Burn out after pushing the boundaries of work and play too far	- Symptoms follow a period of high stress with unhelpful coping strategies backfiring (e.g. over-reliance on caffeine, alcohol etc.) - Digestive havoc, headaches and erratic sleep pattern	- Lack of sleep - Mental stress and pressure - On waking - Background noise	- Later in the day - Getting a good nights sleep - Passing a stool - Peace and quiet	**Nux vomica**
Physical burn out with severe muscle aches all over the body	- This remedy is most useful when former couch potatoes take up a very challenging exercise regime - Muscle aches are combined with exhaustion and tiredness that is intensified by not being able to sleep comfortably at night	- Sudden jolting movements - After a sleep - Being touched or hugged	- Resting in a comfortable position	**Arnica**
Strong sense of physical exhaustion with erratic appetite and craving for alcohol	- Follows a period of unhealthy eating - Energy levels plummet and lead to sugar cravings	- Getting too hot - After a hot bath - Standing for a long time - Mid-morning	- Resting - Walking for a short time - Contact with a cool breeze	**Sulphur**

grief

This complex and powerful emotion can be a response to any number of life events that involve a deep sense of loss. The most profound grief is usually in response to the death of a loved one and yet this feeling can also emerge after the break up of a relationship or as a result of experiencing serious and uninitiated changes in lifestyle and circumstances. In fact, grief in some form can accompany any situation that involves a sense of being bereft in its broadest sense.

While everyone experiences their own sense of grief in their own personal way, there are specific stages of the grieving process that enact the natural movement towards emotional healing. The stages are likely to move from shock through to denial, despair, anger and guilt and it's not at all uncommon for the acute phase of distress to be followed by a sense of emotional numbness, depression and/or anxiety as the reality of loss begins to sink in. As recovery progresses, these feelings should gradually occur less frequently and, as more positive emotions emerge, for proportionally longer phases. A sense of being able to take pleasure in life once again should slowly form, although episodes of sadness, wistfulness and depression will still occasionally break through at intervals. These are often triggered by anniversaries and family gatherings or a piece of music on the radio with powerful emotional associations but trivial things can also suddenly and devastatingly catch you unaware, such as seeing someone in the street who resembles the person you have lost.

Symptoms of grief can vary in intensity and frequency but any of the following would be natural part of the process of coming to terms with loss:

- **Sleep disturbance**
- **Mood swings**
- **Emotional withdrawal and flatness**
- **A sense of unreality about what's happened**
- **Random feelings of panic**
- **Emotional, mental and physical exhaustion**
- **Bouts of involuntary weeping**
- **Mental and physical restlessness**
- **Emotional short fuse**
- **Lack of mental focus and concentration**
- **Lack of appetite, food cravings or comfort eating**

It does help to bear in mind that treatment isn't automatically needed for the symptoms of grieving unless they are interfering with your ability to move on with life. If you do feel that you are stuck in one stage of grief, this is exactly the sort of situation that can be assisted by complementary medical support.

From a conventional medical perspective, support is available through grief counselling, and/or medication, such as the short-term use of tranquillisers or antidepressants. Any of the complementary strategies suggested below can be used safely in combination with any prescribed conventional treatment.

practical self-help

❧ Sleeplessness is one of the most common reactions to bereavement and therefore nights can seem interminably long and difficult, often making mood swings worse during the following day. For advice on how to get a wayward sleep pattern back on track, see the section on 'Changes in Sleep Pattern and Sleep Quality' on page 99.

❧ Rescue Remedy can greatly ease the initial shock and trauma of bereavement. Spray it directly on the tongue or dilute a few drops in a small glass of water and sip as often as is required.

❧ Although friends and family can be very supportive and attentive in the immediate stage after bereavement, it helps to be prepared for the phase when they need to get on with their lives once again. If you feel isolated and in need of a good listener, talk to your doctor about the possibility of grief counselling as this service helps those in the process of grieving to voice painful feelings and find strategies for learning how to cope and move on with their lives.

❧ Give yourself enough space within which to grieve, rather than feeling that you have to dash straight back into normal life with a stiff upper lip. Although re-establishing familiar boundaries can help at the right time, brushing painful feelings aside can lead to later complications with anxiety and/or depression.

❧ Although eating well often occupies a very low position on the list of essential things to do in a time of crisis, this is the very time when you are going to receive essential benefit from this kind of sustenance. Vitamins are particularly important, especially vitamin B which supports the nervous system, so eat plenty of wholegrains, unroasted, unsalted nuts, green leafy vegetables, fish, yeast extract, brown rice, bananas and products made from soya flour.

❧ Spritzing the face with a diluted solution of orange blossom or rose water can feel emotionally re-balancing and uplifting.

❧ Using five or six drops of ylang ylang, clary sage, geranium, or lavender essential oils in a warm bath can feel comforting at the end of an emotionally challenging day. Alternatively, any of these can be vaporised in an essential oil burner to create a soothing environment.

❧ Sipping an infusion of chamomile or lemon balm can help ease some of the initial symptoms of shock that accompany bereavement. Chamomile has the added benefit of helping to calm and relax the mind and body when taken before going to bed.

CAUTION!

IF ANY OF THE FOLLOWING OCCUR, CONSULT YOUR DOCTOR:

• Symptoms of grief that refuse to move on, or appear to be getting worse as time goes by

• Signs and symptoms of lingering or escalating depression. See the previous section on 'Mild to Moderate Depression' on page 231 for a check list of the potential symptoms to watch out for

TYPE OF GRIEF	GENERAL SYMPTOMS	WORSE FROM	BETTER FOR	REMEDY NAME
Classic grief symptoms with frequent bouts of uncontrollable weeping	- Moods alternate between tears and laughter - Lots of sighing and/or muscle tension and twitching - This remedy is equally helpful in the first stage and more established phases of grief when these symptoms are present	- Shock - Touch - Becoming chilled - Coffee - Smoking - Yawning	- Eating small amounts often - Being alone - Taking relaxing, regular, deep breaths - Firm pressure	**Ignatia**
Severe anxiety that follows hearing bad news	- This remedy can be especially helpful in the very first stage of grief when the news has come as a great shock - It can also help the fear and panic that follows after witnessing a traumatic incident	- Touch - At night - Noisy surroundings	- Fresh air - Moderate warmth - Rest	**Aconite**
Later stages of suppressed grief with an inability to cry	- Painful feelings are pushed below the surface - Aversion to sympathy and fuss due to a fear of being humiliated by crying in front of anyone - Avoids company for this reason	- Affection - Being touched - After crying - Becoming overheated - Noise	- Cool, fresh air - Rest - Being given some peace and quiet	**Natrum mur**
Later stages of grief with a huge need for comfort and sympathy	- Clingy, weepy and in need of a lot of sensitive care and attention - Symptoms get more distressing when feeling isolated	- In the evening and at night - When resting - In bed - Getting hot and bothered	- Taking gentle exercise - Contact with fresh, cool air - Affection - After a cry	**Pulsatilla**
Angry stage of grief	- This remedy can be very helpful in resolving symptoms that are a result of suppressed anger - Physical and mental oversensitivity leads to a tendency to become disproportionally angry over trivial matters	- Excitement - Becoming chilled - During the night - Feeling stressed	- After breakfast - Resting - Warmth	**Staphysagria**

homeopathy

lack of concentration

This is a frustrating problem that tends to be at its worst when high stress levels are poorly managed. Escalating background pressure distracts the mind, making it extremely difficult to focus effectively on the job at hand. Additional triggers can include any of the following:

- **Depression**
- **Pre-menstrual syndrome**
- **Anxiety**
- **Lack of good quality sleep**
- **Hormonal changes**
- **Unstable blood sugar levels**
- **Inappropriate stress-deflecting measures such as drinking too much alcohol**

Everyone is likely to go through phases of being less than 100 per cent sharp and this need not be a problem if it occurs for an obvious reason and improves quickly. However, if you frequently feel not quite on the ball, it is worth addressing the underlying causes. The conventional medical approach would consider diagnoses of anxiety, depression, diabetes or a hormone imbalance and, if necessary, treat with beta-blockers, antidepressants, blood sugar balancing formulations (combined with dietary advice), or hormone therapy. If no underlying medical conditions can be detected, behavioural techniques, such as a stress management plan, may be suggested.

From a complementary medical perspective there's a great deal that can be done to help restore mental focus and concentration that's the result of high, poorly managed stress levels. However, if one of the underlying conditions mentioned above is confirmed, help from a complementary source will need to be supervised by an experienced practitioner.

practical self-help

❧ Keep blood sugar levels stable by eating regular, small snacks of whole grain products combined with a small portion of protein. Kick the caffeine habit and substitute with green tea as this has a lower caffeine yield but will still give you a lift.
❧ Zinc plays an important part in mental focus and memory enhancement so include seeds, beans, nuts, fish, oysters, meat and lentils in your diet. There have been a few safety concerns regarding zinc supplements so it is preferable to source it nutritionally.
❧ Meditating on a daily basis can help you switch off the constant background chatter that goes on in a typically stressed mind and will allow you to focus with greater clarity and mental energy on whatever tasks are in front of you.

✹ Make a regular, refreshing night's sleep a priority. Dreaming sleep plays a vital role in allowing psychological conflicts to be safely worked through while you are resting and, when this is undisturbed, you can face the next day feeling focused and clear-headed. Sleep deprivation, on the other hand, can lead to mental confusion and disorientation.

✹ Vaporise peppermint, rosemary, grapefruit and lemon essential oils in a burner or place a single drop on a tissue and inhale as often as is necessary to clear the mind.

CAUTION!

Seek immediate medical advice if mental confusion and lack of focus is accompanied by slurred speech and numbness in the limbs

TYPE OF LACK OF CONCENTRATION	GENERAL SYMPTOMS	WORSE FROM	BETTER FOR	REMEDY NAME
Lack of mental focus from anticipating stress	- This is great for anticipatory worries about an imminent major event that are distracting you from the task at hand - Once the pressure is on and it's time to perform, mental focus slips back into gear	- Thinking about stress - In the middle of the afternoon - Indigestible foods	- Gentle exercise - Loosening restrictive clothing - Meeting a challenge	**Lycopodium**
Poor concentration from lack of sound, refreshing sleep	- Ongoing, high stress levels lead to a reliance on caffeine to keep up the pace and alcohol to to unwind - Irritable and jittery with hangover-type headache made worse from poor quality sleep - Combination of muzzy-headedness with feeling like a coiled spring	- On first waking - Disruptive surroundings - Lack of rest - Eating badly and irregularly	- Peaceful, relaxed surroundings - As the day goes on - Making time for sound sleep	**Nux vomica**

materia medica (remedy profiles)

This section includes the majority of the homeopathic remedies common to family prescribing that are indicated throughout the book and aims to give you a grasp of the multi-faceted features or 'personality' of each remedy. As you become more familiar with this information you will be able to recognise the homeopathy labels on the shelves at your local health food shop or pharmacy and select whichever is appropriate for your needs with confidence.

aconite

Made from the bluish-violet Monkshood plant, Aconite is often indicated for: the initial stages of anxiety; chicken pox; croup; earaches; fevers; measles; palpitations; panic attacks; shock; sore throats and teething.

Core Features
• Any condition that comes on rapidly as a result of exposure to dry, cold winds
• Restlessness
• Problems often caused by waking during the night
• Extreme sensitivity to pain and discomfort
• Severe chilliness with twitchiness and tense muscles

N.B. This remedy is most useful in the first stage of any bout of inflammation or infection (within the first 24–48 hours). When well indicated, symptoms should clear up as quickly as they appeared.

Emotional State
• Panic comes on very quickly and violently when unwell, to the point of fearing that death must be imminent. (This is a common feature of panic attacks in anyone who hasn't experienced them before)
• Feelings of panic aggravated by crowds, big open spaces and the dark
• Hypersensitive and hyper-reactive to all impressions
• Extreme emotional reactions to general shock or trauma

Head
• Emotionally upsetting or traumatic events bring on sudden headaches accompanied by dizziness
• Headaches go together with the fever that's associated with the early stages of inflammation (e.g. the early stages of a cold or ear infection)
• Head pains are relieved by contact with fresh air and become worse in stuffy, overheated rooms
• Headaches triggered by a blocked nose are relieved by fresh air, provided it's not too cold and biting
• Although lying down and trying to rest aggravates most other symptoms, it specifically relieves headaches and dizziness

Eyes
• Problems with eyes develop dramatically and suddenly
• Eyes feel sore and watery and look bloodshot after exposure to dry, cold winds, or after reflection of sunlight on snow
• Eye injuries with burning pains and swelling around the eye socket

Respiratory (Nose, Throat and Chest)
• Runny nose with clear discharge after exposure to dry, cold winds
• Nasal discharge feels hot and burning
• Dry, tingling sensation in the throat makes it uncomfortable to swallow
• Sensations of constriction in the throat are combined with redness and rapid-developing inflammation
• Dry, croupy cough is brought on after a chill
• Anxious breathlessness is worse during sleep or on waking
• Cough disturbs sleep with choking sensation that exaggerates feelings of anxiety and terror
• Anxiety palpitations and feeling generally feverish and flustered

Ears
• Earaches come on fast and hard after exposure to dry, cold winds, causing a sense of restlessness and distress

Fever
• High temperatures follow unprotected exposure to sharp,

dry winds or any general chill
• Temperature goes up dramatically and quickly with flushes of heat and a hot head with a cool body
• Hot flushes and night sweats can be triggered by severe fear and anxiety

Digestive

• Stomach and bowel upsets come on quickly after a traumatic experience
• When the digestive tract is upset, everything except water tastes bitter
• Rapidly-developing diarrhoea is accompanied by a marked thirst
• Incredibly restless and sensitive to stomach pains and cramps

Urination

• Retention of urine in newborn babies as a reaction to birth trauma
• Rapidly developing cystitis symptoms with sharp, tearing pains and a constant urge to pass water
• Urine looks concentrated and feels hot when it's being passed

Reproductive

• Menstrual problems that date from a traumatic event
• Cramping pains are associated with hot flushes and a general hypersensitivity to pain
• Anxiety and panic with heavy, bright red, gushing bleeding

Sleep

• Symptoms have a tendency to strike on waking
• Restless, fitful sleep at night triggers drowsiness and lethargy during the day
• Nightmares or insomnia follow being involved in, or witnessing a traumatic incident

SYMPTOMS ARE TRIGGERED OR MADE WORSE BY:

• Exposure to cold, dry, Easterly winds
• Experiencing a severe fright or shock
• Extreme changes of temperature

SYMPTOMS ARE EASED BY:

• Falling into a sound sleep
• Moderate temperatures that don't overheat or chill
• Breaking into a sweat

apis

Apis is prepared from the common hive honey bee and is one of the first remedies to consider for rosy pink swellings and inflammation that develop suddenly. It is often indicated for: allergic reactions; bites and stings; cystitis; fluid retention; heat rash; hives; joint pain and swelling; mumps and measles; nappy rash; sore throats and sunburn.

Core Features

• Rapidly developing rosy pink swellings that look waterlogged under the skin and retain the indent of a finger for a long time after light pressure has been applied
• Extreme sensitivity to heat with stinging pains
• Sensitivity to touch and pressure around the puffy areas

Emotional State

• Fussy, fidgety and irritable
• Symptoms set in as a result of shock, stress or emotional upset
• Difficult to please; demands attention but then rejects it
• Hypersensitive and emotional with a tendency to burst into tears

Head

• Throbbing pains and a sense of having a hot head
• Pains are aggravated by sudden, jarring movements and contact with heat in any form
• Thick, dizzy feeling in the head is relieved by firm pressure and gentle movement

Eyes

• Pink, puffy swellings under the eyes look waterlogged
• Swelling and discomfort are eased by cool bathing and compresses
• Sensitivity to light, which makes eyes water

Respiratory (Nose, Throat and Chest)

• Throat feels constricted and swollen and looks pink and slightly glossy on examination. Swelling includes the uvula (the 'little tongue' that hangs at the back of the throat)
• Inflamed throat makes swallowing even liquids very difficult
• Lots of violent sneezing with allergies like hayfever
• Nostrils either feel constantly blocked, or produce a scanty amount of mucus
• Croupy cough that's eased by raising mucus
• Breathlessness aggravated in warm, stuffy surroundings
• Harsh, dry coughing spasms begin with a tight, constricted feeling in the throat

Ears

• Look red and swollen

Fever

• High fever with noticeable lack of thirst
• Once the fever breaks, thirst kicks in
• Distress and discomfort is made worse for contact with warmth of any kind

Digestive

• Sneezing makes pain and discomfort in stomach more intense

Urination

- Concentrated urine that burns as it's being passed (although there's little in the bladder, there's a frequent urge to pass small amounts)
- Puffy look to the skin around the eyes with associated bladder or kidney problems
- Lack of thirst with bladder problems

Reproductive

- Right-sided ovarian pains that either stay on this side or move to the left

Sleep

- Tosses, turns and may cry out in restless sleep

Joints

- Severe, rapidly-developing stinging in joints that look swollen and puffy
- Chilly hands and feet with inflamed, red fingers and toes
- Painful joints look pink and feel tight

SYMPTOMS ARE TRIGGERED OR MADE WORSE BY:

- Bites and/or stings
- Resting
- Getting too hot
- During the night
- Warm drinks

SYMPTOMS ARE EASED BY:

- Cool compresses, cool bathing or contact with cool air
- Sitting up or getting out of bed and moving around
- Taking gentle exercise

argentum nit

Made from pure crystals of silver nitrate, this remedy is commonly indicated for: anticipatory anxiety; diarrhoea; excess wind; headaches and sleep problems related to an escalation of anxiety and/or stress; and an upset, acid stomach.

Core Features

- Poor coordination with trembling when stressed and anxious
- A general or localised sense of constriction
- Sugar cravings
- Pains are sharp and splinter-like, wherever they occur in the body
- A tendency to ulcers when under pressure and stress

Emotional State

- Incredibly agitated and chatty when tense and anxious
- Anxiety is made much worse when in a crowd, a confined space or looking down from a height
- A tendency to rush at things and do them in double-quick time when depressed
- Constantly fearful of being late and missing appointments
- Dwells on anxious thoughts that results in extreme and exhausting restlessness

Head

- Enlarged, tight feeling with headaches that is soothed by applying firm pressure
- Throbbing pains in the head are intensified by warmth and temporarily eased by contact with cool

Throat

- Constricted feeling in the throat with thick mucus production
- Sticking sensation that feels like a splinter in the throat when swallowing
- Throat and uvula look dark red and inflamed

Fever

- Sense of chill when feeling queasy

Digestive

- Triggered by thinking about a coming stressful event
- Craves sugary foods and cheese, which both make digestive uneasiness worse
- Stomach pain starts in a specific spot but then begins to radiate in all directions
- Unusual symptom of nausea; queasiness is soothed by sour food or drink
- Nausea is temporarily relieved by eating but not eased at all by passing wind
- Small amounts of vomit wash up into the throat when belching
- Noisy wind travels upwards and/or downwards with noticeable distention and bloating
- Diarrhoea from nerves or constipation that alternates with diarrhoea, with a shivering sensation in the bowels

Urinary

- Sharp, sticking pain that moves from the kidneys (at the sides or the mid-back) to the bladder
- Pains feel more intense for being touched, breathing deeply and any kind of movement
- Passing small amounts of concentrated urine causes scalding sensation during and after urinating
- Traces of blood in urine
- Urinary symptoms are brought on by stress and/or anxiety

Reproductive

- Sticking, splintering pains around entrance to vagina with any condition that causes irritation and inflammation, such as thrush
- Painful, irregular periods, experiencing the worst symptoms before and during menstruation
- Ovarian pains with discomfort

radiating from the bottom of the spine to the thighs
- Stomach upset and pain with periods

Sleep
- Finds it impossible to sleep when thinking about a coming stressful event
- Restless, fitful night's sleep leads to achiness on waking
- Can't get comfortable in bed due to cramping pains and feeling either too hot or too cold

SYMPTOMS ARE TRIGGERED OR MADE WORSE BY:
- Thinking about stressful issues
- Stuffy, overheated rooms
- Sugary foods and drinks
- During the night

SYMPTOMS ARE EASED BY:
- Exposure to fresh, cold air that doesn't chill
- Firm pressure

arnica

Made from a homeopathic dilution of the yellow flowering Arnica plant (commonly known as Leopard's bane), this remedy is frequently indicated for: bruises; dental work (not including wisdom tooth extraction); the early stages of a boil or abscess; minor falls and accidents; muscle cramps; muscle pain and stiffness after exercising; pre- and post-operative trauma; the shock and pain that follow a fracture; sprains and strains; vaginal bruising after childbirth and varicose veins.

Core Features
- Bruised, aching pains after trauma or overexertion
- Pains trigger extreme restlessness when trying to relax
- Extreme sensitivity to touch
- Easy bruising
- General sensation of weariness and stiffness

Emotional State
- Feeling shocked after a minor accident takes the form of insisting everything is fine and acting as though nothing has happened
- An aversion to being touched or approached leads to turning down all offers of help. Insists on being left alone and not fussed over
- Restless, agitated and extremely irritable with pain
- Mental and physical oversensitivity with sore, aching muscles
- Withdrawn and depressed with acute pain
- Loss of confidence after an accident or trauma

Head
- Very sharp pain on one side of the head with nausea
- Dizzy on waking

Eyes
- Early stage of a black eye with tenderness of the eye socket and discolouration before the bruise develops

Nose
- Tenderness, swelling and/or bleeding from the nose after an injury

Digestive
- Nausea with increased production of saliva, especially at the thought of eating
- Wind in the abdomen with colicky, spasmodic pains

Urination
- Although there's a desire to urinate, has to wait a while before the flow of urine starts; often happens after strenuous exercise
- Frequent urge to pass water, which is only done with great effort and difficulty

Reproductive
- Bruised pains after childbirth cause great distress at night

Flushes
- Frequent, exhausting hot flushes during the menopause that affect the head, while the body feels cold and clammy

Sleep
- Wakeful and restless at night due to aching muscles making it impossible to find a comfortable spot in bed
- Light, fitful sleep with a tendency to nightmares

Joints and Muscles
- Muscular overexertion triggers generalised aching and throbbing
- Aching in the arms and legs leads to an overall feeling of weariness and exhaustion
- Sore, bruised pains are accompanied by swelling in the early stages of sprains and strains

Skin
- Painful, drawing sensations in skin where a boil or abscess is forming, but hasn't yet come to a head
- Tenderness, aching and swelling of traumatised tissue

SYMPTOMS ARE TRIGGERED OR MADE WORSE BY:
- Physical trauma of any kind
- Strenuous physical exercise
- Jarring movement
- Damp, cold conditions
- Fuss and attention when upset
- Overexposure to heat and sunlight

SYMPTOMS ARE EASED BY:
- Resting with the head slightly lower than the body

arsenicum album

Made from a white oxide of metallic arsenic, this remedy is useful for treating: anxiety; chicken pox; colds; cystitis; diarrhoea; dry, inflamed skin; dry, tickly coughs; flu; hayfever; heartburn; indigestion; mild to moderate depression; morning sickness; nappy rash; period pain; sleep disturbance and vomiting.

Core Features
- Burning pains that are soothed by contact with warmth
- Extreme restlessness, particularly at night
- Marked chilliness but with a desire for fresh air on the head and face
- Vomiting and diarrhoea that occur together

Emotional State
- Restless and anxious, especially at night
- Although exhausted, still gets upset about messy environments and won't relax until everything is tidy
- Obsessive fears about health, cleanliness, germs and death
- Loses hope that getting well again is possible
- Fear of losing control is central to anxiety and distress
- Very critical of oneself and others: exceptional high standards are often impossible to achieve

Head
- This is the only part of the body that feels much improved for contact with cool, fresh air
- Headaches have a pattern of developing in the afternoon and building steadily as the night goes on
- Common headache triggers include anxiety and tension, or becoming overheated

Eyes
- Sore, burning, bloodshot eyes are incredibly sensitive to bright light

Respiratory (Nose, Throat and Chest)
- Scanty, clear, burning discharge from the nose makes the skin around the nostrils feel sore and inflamed
- Lots of violent sneezing that causes the nose to run
- Throat feels tight and burning and is temporarily relieved by taking small sips of warm drinks
- Tight sensation in the chest with a dry, tickly, wheezy cough
- Coughing spasms are more intense at night when lying down
- Wheezing and coughing are brought on or made more intense by anxiety and stress

Ears
- Severe tingling, itching and/or burning in the ears

Fever
- Incredibly chilly with a craving for warmth that provides a sense of comfort
- Thirst for small sips of warm, soothing drinks
- Although burning up, feels as though waves of ice-cold water are rippling through the body

Digestive
- Can't stand the thought or sight of food because nausea is so strong
- Exhausted due to suffering diarrhoea and vomiting together
- Burning pains in stomach are temporarily soothed by sipping a warm drink, or placing a warm compress on the affected area
- When vomiting is a problem, cold drinks are thrown up almost straight away
- Diarrhoea is profuse, watery and feels burning as it is passed

Urination
- Kidney or bladder infections lead to a general sense of being feverish, chilly and exhausted
- Burning pains on passing urine cause great distress
- Dehydration can occur as a result of kidney infection with periodical vomiting and a high fever

Reproductive
- Severe period cramps that cause vomiting and/or diarrhoea
- Extreme restlessness with period pain that makes the overall sense of exhaustion worse
- Cramps are noticeably eased by holding a hot water bottle against the painful area and/or soaking in a warm bath
- Severe cramps cause great distress at night

Sleep
- Severe physical and mental restlessness at night makes it very difficult to get a refreshing night's sleep
- Wakes in the early hours feeling anxious and gets up to make a warm drink
- Drowsy by day and wakeful at night
- Anxious thoughts about all that needs to be done the next day make sleep impossible

Skin
- Dry, burning, itchy patches of skin that feel temporarily eased by warmth
- Compulsive scratching makes the skin raw and sometimes causes weeping
- Rubbing temporarily eases the itching, but the burning sensation remains

SYMPTOMS ARE TRIGGERED OR MADE WORSE BY:
- Becoming chilled
- In the dark
- After midnight
- Lying flat
- Cold drinks
- Alcohol

SYMPTOMS ARE EASED BY:

• Exposure of the head to fresh air while the body is kept comfortably warm
• Warmth in general
• Sipping a warm drink
• Being distracted
• Gentle movement that doesn't exhaust
• Breaking into a sweat

belladonna

Made from the entire belladonna plant just as it comes into flower, this remedy can be useful in treating: boils; chicken pox; croup; earache; the first stages of a cold or flu; headaches; high temperatures; hot flushes; mastitis; migraines; mild sunburn; mild sunstroke; mumps; nappy rash; sore throats and teething.
Like Aconite, this remedy is most likely to help in the first stages of a condition (eg the feverish stage of a cold, or the first twinge of earache). You can expect a quick, positive reaction; improvement within minutes rather than hours.

Core Features

• Conditions develop abruptly and dramatically
• Inflammation with dry, bright red skin that radiates a strong sensation of heat
• Symptoms are characteristically right-sided, or worse on the right than the left
• Pains are throbbing and pounding
• Hypersensitivity with marked irritability
• Temperature rises quickly and dramatically

Emotional State

• Very irritable and easily put out when unwell
• Normally placid, easygoing personalities become demanding, and difficult to please
• Easily startled and over-excited
• Restless and agitated, but not as fearful as those who need Aconite
• Wants to be left in peace when unwell
• Alternation between extreme lethargy and excitability

Head

• Fast-developing throbbing headache with very sensitive scalp
• Discomfort and pain are temporarily eased by bending the head backwards
• Right-sided headaches with wooziness that are worse for any kind of movement
• Sensual stimulation of any kind makes pain more intense

Eyes

• Inflamed, bloodshot eyes that feel hot, gritty and watery
• Twitchy eyelids
• Eyes look glassy with large pupils (often associated with a high temperature)
• Throbbing pains in eye sockets with severe headache; this may be more intense on the right side

Ears

• Right-sided throbbing earache that comes on quickly and violently
• Sharp, piercing pains with the outer ear looking red and feeling very hot
• Very sensitive to noise

Respiratory (Throat, Nose and Chest)

• Tonsils get quickly inflamed and throbbing pains affect the throat and glands – may be more noticeable on the right side
• Swallowing is very difficult due to the degree of dryness and swelling in the throat
• Fast-developing hoarseness that can lead to complete loss of voice
• Hot, flushed face with inflammation at the tip of the nose
• Coughing spasms begin with irritation and tickling sensation in the throat
• Barking, croupy cough that is more noticeable when lying in bed at night

Fever

• Sudden onset of fever that rises very dramatically with a rapid pulse rate
• Skin looks bright red and feels hot and dry
• Extreme sensitivity to cold air draughts
• Dry flushes cause the skin to turn bright red, but it remains dry and hot rather than clammy

Digestive

• Thirst for citrus-flavoured drinks
• Very sensitive to taste
• Spasmodic stomach cramps are temporarily eased by bending forwards or backwards but light touch causes distress
• Diarrhoea with constant urge to empty the bowels

Urination

• Urine looks cloudy, bloody or dark with kidney or bladder infection
• Urinating is very painful, with a burning, cutting sensation
• Spasms in the bladder after passing water
• Incontinence becomes more of a problem when walking or standing for an extended period of time

Reproductive

• Right-sided ovarian pain and discomfort
• Flooding, bright-red menstrual flow with painful cramps
• Cramping pains are especially severe before small clots are passed
• Bearing down feeling in the pelvis

Skin

- Dry, sunburnt skin: surface of the skin radiates heat

SYMPTOMS ARE TRIGGERED OR MADE WORSE BY:

- Too much exposure to sun or bright light
- Uncovering
- Light touch or lying on sensitive areas
- Noisy surroundings
- Sudden, jarring movements

SYMPTOMS ARE EASED BY:

- Moderate warmth
- Bending the head backwards
- Uninterrupted rest
- Lying propped up in a dark room
- Peace and quiet

bryonia

Made from the White Bryony plant, which has bright green leaves and black berries and is a very common sight in the English countryside, this remedy is often used to treat: acute joint pains; constipation; croup; dry, tickly coughs; flu; haemorrhoids; headaches; indigestion; insomnia; the later stages of sprains and muscle strains; mastitis; measles; mumps and whooping cough.

Core Features

- Dryness is the main characteristic of this remedy and is particularly associated with the mucus membranes in the mouth and nose, and the synovial capsules in the joints
- Inflammatory pain is aggravated by even the slightest movement
- Symptoms progress slowly (in contrast to conditions that escalate dramatically and that respond well to Aconite or Belladonna)
- Symptoms that involve the lungs, such as dry tickly coughs that are associated with muscle pain in the chest
- All symptoms are aggravated (or triggered) by low-grade dehydration

Emotional State

- Symptoms may be a result of suppressed anger
- Difficult to please and on an emotional short fuse, especially if sleep patterns have recently been disrupted
- Frustrated and angry about feeling unwell
- Intolerant and flies off the handle when contradicted
- During illness, anxiety focuses on financial worries

Head

- Throbbing headaches often go together with feeling generally 'toxic' as a result of persistent constipation
- Pain is temporarily eased by applying pressure to the spot, or keeping the head very still
- Bursting pains tend to be located above the eyes (the right side may feel more intense) or at the back of the head and feel worse for bending over

Eyes

- Grittiness, dryness and burning are aggravated by movement and any contact with heat

Ears

- Extreme sensitivity to sharp, cold winds
- Ears either feel blocked or hearing is very sensitive to noise

Respiratory (Nose, Throat and Chest)

- Nose feels dry and sore and looks very red and inflamed
- Dryness in the nose and throat creates a general sense of irritation and discomfort
- Pain in the forehead is linked to nasal congestion
- Dry, tickly cough that begins with irritation in the throat
- Persistent dry cough that fails to raise any mucus off the chest
- Coughing spasms that are triggered by walking into a warm environment
- Constant sense of wanting to take a deep breath but this aggravates the cough

Fever

- Obvious dislike of being too wrapped up, especially in warm surroundings
- Fever breaks into a sweat at night
- Thirst for long drinks of cold water

Digestive

- Nausea and queasiness with heavy feeling in the stomach that feels worse for even the slightest movement but is temporarily relieved by belching
- Dry mouth with thirst for cold drinks
- Stomach feels very tender and sore
- Diarrhoea may be brought on by eating too much tart, acid fruit
- Stubborn constipation with dry, hard stools that are very difficult to pass (probably triggered by low-grade dehydration)

Urination

- Burning sensation before passing concentrated urine that feels hot as it leaves the bladder
- Incontinence, triggered by stress, is worse for lifting heavy weights

Reproductive

- Very sore breasts with pre-menstrual syndrome; especially painful for even the slightest movement
- Delayed period as a result of high stress levels or a phase of unusually strenuous physical effort
- Engorged breasts that feel hot and painful

Sleep

- Drowsy during the day due to poor quality sleep at night
- Finds it difficult to mentally switch off at night and/or wakes during the night feeling anxious
- Fitful sleep can lead to recurrent nightmares or episodes of sleepwalking

Joints and Muscles

- Acutely painful, hot swollen joints that feel taut
- Sharp, tearing pains that feel worse for even the slightest movement
- Intense sense of restlessness, even though movement is uncomfortable
- Walking is a problem due to aching and soreness in the feet and/or weakness in the thigh muscles
- Established stage of sprains and strains where the affected area feels better for resting in bed but becomes increasingly painful throughout the day

SYMPTOMS ARE TRIGGERED OR MADE WORSE BY:

- Getting moving after rest
- Overdoing mental and/or physical effort
- Warmth
- Becoming dehydrated

SYMPTOMS ARE EASED BY:

- Keeping as still as possible
- Firm pressure
- Breaking into a sweat
- Cold drinks and cool surroundings

calc carb

Made from Calcium carbonate, derived from the interior of an oyster shell, this remedy can be helpful in treating: chilblains; cradle cap; dry, chapped skin; hot flushes and night sweats; nappy rash; painful teething and thrush. This is a remedy that is deep-acting and is often used by homeopaths to treat ongoing, chronic complaints. It can still be well indicated for some short-term, acute conditions, but in this context it will require far less repetition than Aconite or Belladonna.

Core Features

- Metabolism feels sluggish with noticeable weight gain
- Persistent fatigue with very poor physical stamina
- Constantly chilly and sweaty: perspiration may have a sour smell
- The whole body feel sluggish with circulatory disorders, digestive discomfort and difficulty maintaining mental focus
- Recurrent problems with sprained or strained joints and muscles due to lack of ligament and muscle tone
- Recurrent minor infections such as colds, sore throats and ear infections
- With babies and infants, developmental milestones are late e.g. teething, closure of fontanelles (the soft spot at the crown of the head that's open in newborns), walking and talking
- Poor calcium absorption leads to a high risk of osteoporosis

Emotional State

- Insecurity and poor self-esteem originate from childhood
- Lack of confidence produces a strong dislike of being the centre of attention
- Very nervous and sensitive by nature; specific fears and phobias include anxiety in the dark and when alone
- Tasks need to be done slowly and methodically or otherwise thinking clearly is made impossible as a result of feeling under pressure or rushed
- Becomes withdrawn, stubborn and obstinate in response to feeling threatened and insecure
- Capacity for great conscientiousness when tasks are done at a suitable steady pace

Head

- Headaches are triggered by too much physical exertion, loud noise, bright light, or exposure to cold winds and chill
- Queasiness associated with headache and dizziness is eased by resting in a comfortably warm room

Eyes

- Eye strain sets in rapidly after reading and watching television

Ears

- Earache with pulsating, shooting pains as a result of exposure to cold winds
- Relapsing episodes of earache with swollen glands in the winter months

Respiratory (Nose, Throat and Chest)

- Recurrent sore throats in the winter with noticeably swollen glands
- Croaky throat on waking or painless loss of voice
- Discomfort and soreness in the nose with a sense of obstruction from thick nasal mucus
- Tickly cough at night
- Coughing spasms raise loose mucus from the chest that looks yellow and tastes sweet
- Coughing spasms make the discomfort of a headache more intense

Fever and Flushes

- A tendency to poor circulation leads to persistently cold, clammy hands and feet and occasional hot, sweaty flushes
- At night the area around the head gets damp and sweaty
- High temperature causes the body to sweat very readily when making even the smallest physical effort
- Hot flushes are triggered by feeling anxious and/or being under physical or mental pressure. They begin with a sensation of burning heat and quickly turn into drenching, clammy sweats

Digestive

- Slow digestion leads to a persistent tendency to indigestion, nausea, and belching that brings up a sour taste into the mouth
- Recurrent constipation or alternation between diarrhoea and constipation with sour-smelling stools
- Aversion to milky, slimy foods such as milk puddings but craves carbohydrates, sweets and also salt
- The peculiar symptom of feeling better when constipated

Urination

- Bladder infections with very concentrated urine that is sour or offensive-smelling

Reproductive

- Pre-menstrual syndrome with severe breast enlargement and tenderness
- A phase of high stress and anxiety can make periods irregular or bring them on early
- Thrush involves the production of thick, burning and sour-smelling discharge, which is aggravated by cravings for sugary food and drink
- Stomach pain accompanies period pain cramps

Sleep

- Children suffer from night terrors, tooth grinding or sleepwalking
- Wakes in the early hours of the morning disturbed and agitated
- Night sweats are common
- Burning hot soles of the feet during the night

Joints and Muscles

- Frequent sprains and strains due to poor muscle tone and ligament fibre
- Ankles are susceptible to injury due to their tendency to 'turn' easily
- Arthritic joints become swollen and painful: a situation aggravated by a tendency to gain weight easily
- Recurrent cramping pain in calf muscles, especially during the night
- Fractures easily, generally in the wrist and ankle joints, as a result of very minor falls or injuries

Skin

- Skin is parched and dry, especially during the cold winter months when chapping and cracking can be a problem
- Babies have a strong tendency to cradle cap and/or nappy rash
- Classic infantile eczema that develops on the face, and inside the flexions (bends) of the elbow and knee

SYMPTOMS ARE TRIGGERED OR MADE WORSE BY:

- Chilly, damp weather
- Major shifts in temperature and weather, especially the transition from warm to chilly
- Being watched when under pressure
- Being forced to do anything at a fast pace

SYMPTOMS ARE EASED BY:

- Resting and generally taking it easy
- Warm, dry weather
- Steady, moderate temperatures

cantharis

Made from a homeopathic dilution of Spanish fly, otherwise known as a blister beetle which is a handsome green colour and is common in southern France and Spain, this remedy can be helpful for: conjunctivitis; cystitis; insect bites; mild sunburn; minor burns and scalds; nappy rash and sore throats.

Core Features

- Stinging, burning pains
- Symptoms tend to develop dramatically and rapidly, and often relapse at intervals. In order to work most effectively, this remedy should be given at the first twinge of discomfort
- A strong sensation of burning up inside can also be accompanied by shivering and chilliness

Emotional State

- Fussy and fidgety when feeling ill
- Drowsy and tired with a raised temperature
- Hyper-responsive to external stimuli such as exposure to bright light or being touched, especially on the throat
- Confused or in a state of extreme excitement when feverish

Head

- Burning, throbbing, or stabbing pains with headaches that often stem from the nape of the neck
- Relief from tension headaches comes from walking or moving about

Eyes

- Smarting and burning sensation with rapidly-developing eye infections such as conjunctivitis

Throat

- Difficulty swallowing even liquids

because of severe swelling in the throat

Fever
- Restless and prostrated with a high temperature
- Face can be very flushed or pale when feverish
- Noticeable clammy sweat on the arms and legs when going through a shivery phase

Urination (This is Cantharsis' major sphere of action)
- Burning, cutting pains in the bladder are felt before, during and after passing water
- Similar pains may be felt higher up in the kidneys
- A general sense of discomfort and tenderness may extend through the whole of the urinary system along with a rapidly developing temperature

Sleep
- Sleepy during the day but disturbed sleep at night caused by the discomfort of symptoms

Skin
- Burning sensation caused by minor domestic burns or too much sun exposure
- Large blisters with burning pains
- Stinging, burning pains with insect bites

SYMPTOMS ARE TRIGGERED OR MADE WORSE BY:
- Sensory stimulation
- Swallowing liquids
- Drinking coffee
- Touching sensitive areas of skin

SYMPTOMS ARE EASED BY:
- Passing wind
- Warmth

carbo veg
This remedy is made from vegetable charcoal, which contains carbon as it has been heated in the absence of oxygen, and can be used to relieve: acidity in the stomach; colic; diarrhoea; fainting; flatulence; headaches; indigestion; loss of voice; minor heat exhaustion and sunstroke; minor shock; nosebleeds; 'tired all the time' syndrome; varicose veins and whooping cough.

Core Features
- Extreme exhaustion and tiredness to the point of collapse
- 'Air hunger' with constant yawning and a craving for fresh air
- Skin looks pale and feels damp, and clammy to the touch
- Burning pains that occur anywhere in the body
- Copes very poorly with adjusting to rapid or marked shifts in temperature
- Generally poor circulation with a tendency to flush, particularly after eating
- Sensation of burning internal heat combined with icy coldness on the surface of the body
- Easy bleeding and/or ulceration of the tissues

Emotional State
- Listless and indifferent
- Irritable and excitable in the evening
- Confused thought patterns with poor memory
- Sad and depressed when feeling ill
- Generally anxious with specific fear of the dark

Head
- Confusion and dizziness with hangover-type headaches
- Tension in the scalp or temples, or as if wearing a tight band around the head
- Head pains radiate to the jaw and ears
- Headaches are brought on by wearing something tight round the head or becoming overtired

Ears
- Blocked sensation in the ears with tinnitus (noises in the ears)
- Ear infections produce swollen glands and a watery or offensive smelling discharge

Respiratory (Nose, Throat and Chest)
- Acute cold symptoms can bring on nosebleeds that ooze rather than gush and are slow to clot
- Colds spread quickly to the throat with burning pain, hoarseness or loss of voice
- Throat symptoms are brought on or made worse by clearing the throat, talking and/or exposure to damp air, especially in the evening
- Tickling or crawling sensation in the throat
- Coughing spasms that lead to gagging or actual vomiting
- Burning sensation in the chest

Fever
- Cold and clammy to the touch but feels burning hot inside
- Although very chilly, feels worse in a heated room and craves fresh, cool air, which relieves
- Drenching sweats break at night and disturb sleep
- Very hot until the sweat breaks, when there is an extreme sense of being chilled to the bone

Digestive
(This remedy can be incredibly helpful in releasing trapped wind that follows investigative tests such as a laparoscopy or barium enema, or any form of abdominal surgery that results in trapped wind.)
- Large amount of trapped wind that causes great discomfort before it's released
- Burning sensation in the stomach with queasiness and

nausea that belching relieves temporarily
- Stomach symptoms follow a period of overindulgence in food and/or alcohol
- Watery diarrhoea results in a feeling of complete exhaustion, with burning pain around the perineal area
- Piles that bleed very easily and quickly after the least amount of straining

Urination
- Urgent need to urinate
- Flow of urine is slow to start after a night's sleep
- Smarting sensation when passing small amounts of urine that is very concentrated looking

Sleep
- Sleep is fitful and twitchy; wakes suddenly bathed in sweat
- Fear of going back to sleep
- Wakes in the morning feeling unrefreshed

Circulation
- Numb feeling in the limbs
- Burning pains in varicose veins
- 'Restless legs' make it difficult to sleep at night

SYMPTOMS ARE TRIGGERED OR MADE WORSE BY:
- Stuffy, airless rooms
- Damp conditions
- After eating
- Becoming chilled
- Drinking alcohol
- Walking out of doors in cold, frosty weather
- During the night

SYMPTOMS ARE EASED BY:
- Being gently fanned
- Contact with fresh, cool air
- Initially after belching
- Falling into a sound sleep

causticum

Made from a homeopathic dilution of equal proportions of slaked lime (calcium hydroxide) to potassium bisulphate, this remedy can be helpful in easing: bladder infections; coughs; minor burns; sore throats with a hoarse voice and stress-related exhaustion.

Core Features
- In contrast to Aconite or Belladonna where acute symptoms sweep up speedily and dramatically, symptoms that respond well to this remedy develop slowly and insidiously
- A slow-developing, progressive sense of being 'run down', often as a result of an extended period of emotional strain or high stress levels
- Marked sense of fatigue and exhaustion with a noticeable desire to rest and take it easy
- Wherever they surface in the body, pains feel sore, burning and cramping
- Stiffness and discomfort in the small joints of the hands and the feet
- Common triggers of illness include exposure to sharp, cold winds, exhaustion, or lack of sleep

Emotional State
- Hyper-emotional with a tendency to be overwrought in response to the slightest excitement
- Lack of mental focus/poor memory as a result of exhaustion
- Anxiety leads to obsessive or compulsive behaviour
- Anxiety is aggravated by being alone in the dark which can develop into a strong fear of going to bed
- Intense sympathy and empathy with injustice shown towards others: may find it hard to establish firm psychological boundaries in order to prevent getting burnt out emotionally
- Hyper-critical of others, sarcastic and short-fused when feeling ill

Head
- Sick and dizzy with headache
- Headaches are combined with neuralgic pains or numbness in the face (often more intense on, or limited to, the right side)

Respiratory (Throat, Nose and Chest)
- Lots of yellow-green mucus at the back of the throat
- Rawness and burning in the throat with complete loss of voice or painful hoarseness, which is worse on waking
- Nose feels itchy and blocked
- Coughing spasms start with a tickling sensation in the throat
- Sipping cold drinks temporarily eases coughing spasms and contact with warm air makes them worse
- Coughing leads to burning, raw sensations in the throat and chest

Digestive
- Extreme thirst for cold drinks
- Burning in the stomach with acid that rises into the throat
- Raw, itching discomfort with piles or anal fissure

Urination
- Stress incontinence is triggered by laughing, sneezing, coughing or excitement
- Marked sensitivity to cold with cystitis
- Desire to pass urine frequently: a large amount is passed each time

Sleep
- Restless legs at night prevent sound sleep
- Anxiety at night: wakes from a fitful sleep with a start

Skin
- Minor burns are slow to heal and remain surprisingly sensitive

Joints and Muscles

• Stiff, swollen joints that
are especially painful on
first movement
• Cramping pains in the calf
muscles and feet

SYMPTOMS ARE TRIGGERED OR MADE WORSE BY:

• Lack of sleep and rest
• Rapid or violent changes
of temperature
• Exposure to cold windy weather
• During the night
• Getting drenched

SYMPTOMS ARE EASED BY:

• Cold drinks
• Warm, humid weather
• Most symptoms are eased by
resting in a warm bed

chamomilla

Made from a homeopathic dilution
of Wild Chamomile, this remedy
is especially well indicated for:
colic; teething problems and
neuralgia and may also be helpful
for: croup; labour pains; mumps;
painful periods; sciatica and
whooping cough.

Core Features

• Extreme mental and emotional
sensitivity leads to temper
tantrums
• Flushed with most conditions
• Marked sense of weakness
with pains
• Whatever symptoms are
presented, they get noticeably
more severe and troublesome
when in bed at night
• Total intolerance of pain
which contributes to a state
of desperation
• Noticeable muscle spasms
and/or twitching
• Symptoms may date from a
phase of unexpressed anger

Emotional State

• In children, irritability reaches
such a crescendo they can't be
distracted or pacified
• Babies and toddlers can only
be pacified and calmed down by
being rocked, carried or driven
for a short distance in the car
• In adults sensitivity to pain
leads to impatience and
frustration, often developing into
an extreme state of intolerance
and irritability
• Noticeable aversion to physical
contact and touch

Head and Face

• Neuralgic pains with associated
pains in the mouth are soothed by
cold (compressed, or holding cold
water in the mouth)
• Headaches are triggered or
aggravated by feeling angry

Ears

• Earache is associated with
generalised swelling of the
glands in the face, jaw and neck
• Bending forwards sets off
shooting pains in the ears

Fever

• Characteristic one-sided flushing
of the face leads to one cheek
glowing red while the other
remains pale (the red cheek is
usually on the most painful side)
• The head and brow become hot
and sweaty with fever

Respiratory (Nose, Throat and Chest)

• Lots of sneezing with a dry
blocked nose, or hot, watery
discharge
• Pain and soreness in the throat
are combined with generalised
glandular swelling and tenderness
• The throat feels tight, making it
uncomfortable to swallow food
• Cough is dry and irritating, with
spasms being triggered by a
tickling sensation behind the
upper part of the breast bone

Digestive

• Severe teething pains are
combined with watery, green-
coloured stools that smell like
rotten eggs
• Bloating after eating with painful
burping
• Colicky pains are temporarily
eased by applying warmth to the
belly: passing wind doesn't provide
any relief

Reproductive

• Dark, clotted flow with period
pains that are so strong they
resemble labour-like contractions
• Periods come early with a
tendency to feel hot, bothered,
cross and feverish with severe
cramps
• Labour contraction pains extend
from the back to the thighs
• Enlarged, incredibly tender
breasts with very sensitive,
sore nipples

SYMPTOMS ARE TRIGGERED OR MADE WORSE BY:

• Windy, draughty and damp
conditions
• Leading up to, or during, periods
• Becoming angry and frustrated
• Coffee
• Lying in bed
• In the first part of the night
• General exposure to heat (as
opposed to local applications)

SYMPTOMS ARE EASED BY:

• Warmth applied locally to painful
area (except for neuralgic pains)
• Being, rocked, carried or driven
• Moist conditions

coffea cruda

Made from a homeopathic dilution of raw coffee berries, this remedy can be especially helpful in easing: migraines; poor sleep quality; tension headaches and stress-related anxiety.

Core Features

- General state of emotional, mental and physical oversensitivity, which leads to a sense of being strung out
- Total intolerance of pain
- Twitchy and shaky
- Moves between a totally 'hyper' state and one of exhaustion

Emotional State

- Torrent of ideas flows through the mind making it almost impossible to mentally focus on one thing
- Pushes boundaries too far, e.g. works on a project until in a state of near burn out
- Severe mood swings: moves from laughter to tears very quickly

Sleep

- Wakeful at night and incredibly sleepy during the day: yawns and stretches constantly
- Insomnia from excitability and an over-active brain
- Hypersensitivity to noise becomes especially acute and distressing at night when attempting to drift off to sleep

Head

- One-sided, sharp headache comes on after waking
- Classic migraine-type headache with a desire to lie down and rest in a darkened room
- Sensation of a rush of blood to the head with a headache

SYMPTOMS ARE TRIGGERED OR MADE WORSE BY:

- Cold
- Contact with fresh air
- Physical contact
- Wine
- Narcotics
- Strong emotion
- During the night

SYMPTOMS ARE EASED BY:

- Lying down
- Warmth

ferrum phos

Made from a homeopathic dilution of Ferric Phosphate, this remedy can be helpful in relieving: borderline anaemia with lethargy; dizziness and/or palpitations; earache and the early stage of a fever.

Core Features

- Chilliness with exhaustion
- Bruised, sore sensations in the muscles
- Symptoms become more intense if sweat doesn't have a chance to break
- Although pale, flushes very easily

Emotional State

- Easily made excitable
- Moods move from being chatty and talkative to withdrawn and exhausted
- Dislikes large crowds
- Poor mental focus leads to frustration

Head

- Dizziness with a general state of weakness
- Hammering headache lodges in temples and forehead
- Headache relieved by a nosebleed

Ears

- Earache with ringing and buzzing in the ears
- Glands in front of the ear become red, sore and swollen

Respiratory (Throat and Chest)

- Painful, sore throat on waking which feels worse when swallowing saliva
- The throat and tonsils look red and inflamed and feel dry
- Laryngitis from over-straining the voice
- Lots of rattling-sounding, green-coloured mucus in the throat and chest
- Coughing spasms are more severe when outside in the fresh air
- Spasms of whooping cough cause retching and vomiting

Fever

- Usually indicated in the first stage of fever with chilliness, exhaustion and aching in the muscles

Urination

- Urine leaks slightly with coughing spasms

SYMPTOMS ARE TRIGGERED OR MADE WORSE BY:

- During the night
- Movement
- Noise
- Jarring movement
- Suppressed sweat
- Becoming chilled

SYMPTOMS ARE EASED BY:

- Onset of a nosebleed
- When lying down
- Cool compresses locally applied

gelsemium

Made from a homeopathic dilution of yellow jasmine (not related to true jasmines, hence its alternative name false jasmine), this remedy can be invaluable when well indicated for: the after-effects of a nasty viral illness (especially the lingering fatigue and mild depression); anticipatory anxiety; dizziness; flu; headaches and migraines; labour pains; measles and painless diarrhoea.

Core Features

- The essence of this remedy can best be summed up by the word 'droopy' whether it applies to the physical, mental or emotional state
- Extreme tiredness with generalised aching in the muscles
- Shivering with chills running up and down the spine
- Shaky and weak limbs from making even the slightest of effort

N.B. This remedy is a 'slow burner' and the kind of symptoms that respond well to it are likely to build slowly and insidiously over a few days. In this sense, it can be regarded as being the opposite of remedies like Aconite and Belladonna that are almost always needed in the first stage of fast-developing acute conditions

Emotional State

- Tired, grumpy and irritable: just wants to be left alone in peace
- Silent, withdrawn anxiety with a tendency to brood quietly
- Extreme mental fatigue
- Indifference and apathy
- Depression is combined with specific fear of the dark and brooding anxiety about death
- Confused and lacking in mental focus
- Symptoms may be triggered by shock or the stressful side of an exhilarating, exciting event

Head

- Headache is like a tight band around the forehead just above the eyes
- Pains may begin by moving from the nape of the neck to the forehead
- Headaches and/or migraines are preceded by dizziness, lack of co-ordination and a general sense of being 'out of it'

Eyes

- Characteristic droopy look to the eyelids accompanies any illness that triggers a washed out feeling
- Blurred vision with dizziness when feeling wobbly and unwell

Respiratory (Nose, Throat and Chest)

- Slow, insidiously-developing cold or flu symptoms that start with a general sense of being unwell, followed by lots of violent sneezing with a hot nasal discharge
- The nose may be uncomfortably blocked with sore inflamed nostrils
- Sense of smell may be incredibly heightened or temporarily lost during a head cold or bout of flu
- Shooting pains with sore throat that travel from the throat to the ears on swallowing
- The throat is typically red and swollen with a sense of a lump
- Severe coughing spasms with sore chest from the muscular effort involved

Fever

- The face and head are hot and feverish with cold arms and legs
- Classic flu picture of feverishness with chills that run up and down the spine with lots of shivering
- Muscles are shaky and tremble with a general sense of wobbliness and weakness when feverish
- Breaking into a sweat doesn't help relieve the fever
- Although uncomfortable and feverish, warmth feels unpleasant rather than comforting

Digestive

- Strange symptom of dry mouth without thirst
- Frequent painless diarrhoea as a result on anticipatory anxiety
- If the diarrhoea is severe, there may be a loss of control to the point of passing an involuntary motion

Reproductive

- Faint and unsteady when pre-menstrual
- Backache contractions with period pains that radiate downwards into the thighs
- The womb feels heavy, pulling downwards during contractions
- Indicated in childbirth for slow dilation of cervix with unproductive contractions, and/or labour pains that settle in the back

Muscles

- General sense of heaviness and weakness in the arms and legs when feeling ill or in pain

SYMPTOMS ARE TRIGGERED OR MADE WORSE BY:

- Getting overheated
- Damp, humid conditions
- Becoming uncomfortably chilled
- Focusing on and thinking about a coming stressful event
- Exposure to bright sunlight

SYMPTOMS ARE EASED BY:

- Keeping surroundings moderately warm
- Contact with fresh air that doesn't chill
- Headaches are specifically eased after passing large quantities of urine

graphites

Made from a homeopathic dilution of black lead, this remedy has a particular affinity with any skin condition that causes inflammation, cracking and weeping of the skin. As a result it's one of the first to think of in cases of: cold sores; impetigo; psoriasis (unusually on the palms of the hands); sore, cracked nipples; thickened nails that crumble easily and weeping eczema.

Core Features

- Sudden onset of weakness and exhaustion for the most minor reasons
- Offensive odour to discharges wherever they appear
- Poor quality, slow healing skin that tends to develop thick, cracked, dry patches, especially in folds of skin
- Sweats as a result of the slightest provocation: tends to smell offensive too
- Gains weight easily with a pale, unhealthy appearance

Head and Face

- Lots of itching on the scalp with a tendency for hair volume and texture to be adversely affected
- Lots of dandruff that responds well to frequent washing: otherwise it builds up
- Sore scalp that feels tender to the touch. This may be due to patches of eczema that have wept and dried into crusts
- Sore, cracked patches at the corners of the lips
- Patches of eczema settle at the sides of the nose and upper lip

Breasts

- Sore and cracked nipples; this is often associated with breast feeding

Skin

- Generally unhealthy skin that becomes infected easily and takes a long time to recover
- Moist eruptions ooze a thick, yellow discharge that dries to a crust-like a glaze
- Cracks and fissures itch and bleed painfully. Areas especially affected are the tips of the fingers, the corners of the mouth, nipples, anus and between the toes
- Burning sensations in old scars
- Nails become thick but brittle; can be a complication of psoriasis

SYMPTOMS ARE TRIGGERED OR MADE WORSE BY:

- Becoming hot in bed
- Exposure to cold to the point of chill
- Damp
- During the night

SYMPTOMS ARE EASED BY:

- When well wrapped up, but allowing for contact with fresh air
- Resting in a dark room

hepar sulph

Made from a homeopathic dilution of an impure form of calcium sulphide, this remedy can be useful in relieving: abcesses; colds in the established stage; coughs; croup; boils; earache; sinusitis; sore throats; styes; swollen glands; tonsilitis and whooping cough.

Core Features

- Discharges, wherever they appear, are characteristically thick and yellowish-green in colour and texture
- Skin is slow to heal and becomes infected quickly
- Discharges smell offensive
- Pains tend to be sharp and splinter-like in nature
- Hypersensitivity on physical, mental and emotional levels with an aversion to getting chilled

Emotional State

- Irritable and reactive; flies off the handle at the slightest provocation
- Intolerant of pain: feels strung out when ill and in discomfort
- May become violent when frustrated and angry
- Grouchy and very hard to please when out of sorts

Eyes

- Hypersensitive to cold air
- Large styes with thick, sticky, yellow discharge (also with conjunctivitis)

Ears

- Earache may lodge in the right ear only, or be more severe on this side

Respiratory (Nose, Throat and Chest)

- Very sensitive sense of smell with a tendency to sneeze on contact with cold air
- Colds come on after getting severely chilled
- Blocked nose: when mucus does appear, it tends to be thick and yellow. There may also be associated sinus congestion, pain and tenderness
- Sore throats with a sensation as though a sharp fish bone were sticking in the side of the throat (this may be noticeably more severe on the right hand side)
- Associated glandular swelling with inflammation of the throat and/or tonsils
- Dry, troublesome cough that is set off or made more intense by inhaling cold air
- Gags and sweats with the effort of bringing up phlegm

Fever

- Very sensitive to, and made uncomfortable by, the slightest draught of cold air

• Perspires heavily when making even the slightest physical effort

Skin

• Large spots, boils and abscesses are slow to come to a head or to resolve themselves
• Quickly infected wounds that are very slow to heal
• Extreme sensitivity to cold air on the surface of the skin

Muscles and Joints

• Joints, especially the knees, are prone to dislocation and feel weak and wobbly when walking
• Stiff, swollen joints are made more uncomfortable for contact with dry, cold air
• Sleep may be disturbed by cramping pains in the thigh and calf muscles

SYMPTOMS ARE TRIGGERED OR MADE WORSE BY:

• Cold drinks and cold food
• Exposure to cold, draughty conditions
• Lying on the painful area
• During the winter months
• In the morning and the evening
• Touching the affected part lightly

SYMPTOMS ARE EASED BY:

• Warmth
• Having something to eat
• Humidity

hypericum

Made from a homeopathic dilution of the plant St John's Wort, this remedy can be very helpful in any of the following situations: after pains of labour; bites and stings; neuralgia; pain that remains at the site of injection; puncture wounds; sensitivity and pain in scar tissue; sciatica and trauma to parts of the body that are especially rich in nerve endings.

Core Features

• Shooting nerve pains
• Hypersensitivity of the affected area, especially to touch
• Pains are more severe and distressing than the extent of the injury would suggest

Emotional State

• Distress or depression following an accident
• In such discomfort that the slightest movement results in weeping

Head

• Hallmark headaches that follow after an injury to the coccyx (base of the spine)
• Neuralgic pains extend into the cheek

Muscles and Joints

• Intermittent shooting pains radiate away from the site of injury (this can also be true of the site of an injection)
• Crushing pains in the fingers, toes and spine following an accident
• Pains are especially severe when rising from a sitting position
• Sciatic pains may be especially severe in, or limited to the left leg
• Muscles tend to jerk and twitch
• Bruised pains in joints
• Intensity of pains makes it difficult to stoop or walk
• Pain feels temporarily relieved from being rubbed

SYMPTOMS ARE TRIGGERED OR MADE WORSE BY:

• Exposure to cold, damp air
• Being touched
• Movement
• In the evening
• In the dark

SYMPTOMS ARE EASED BY:

• Resting the head back
• Keeping as still as possible

ignatia

Referred to as Ignatia amara this remedy is made from a homeopathic dilution of the St Ignatius bean, which is actually the fruit of a plant called Strychnos ignatia. It can be especially helpful in treating: baby blues; bereavement, either in its primary phase, or for later stages of grief; hiccups; lack of appetite or indigestion; muscle tension; sleep problems that date from a period of emotional shock or stress and sore throats (especially if linked with emotional stress or tension).

Core Features

• Symptoms can change rapidly: for instance, laughing one moment and bursting into tears the next
• Unusual, contradictory symptoms such as a sore throat that's eased by swallowing food, or nausea that's relieved by eating
• Repeated sighing, yawning and hiccuping
• Essential aspects of grieving or emotional shock, such as trembling, shaking and/or muscle twitching and tension
• Pains appear and disappear with equal rapidity

N.B. Think imaginatively when considering this as a grief remedy. In other words, apart from providing good emotional support following a death, this remedy can also help someone through the symptoms of grief that emerge even in the absence of a death, such as when a relationship has broken down or when children have grown up and left home, as well as with feelings connected to the end of fertility or the loss of a well-liked job.

Emotional State

• Moods change exhaustingly quickly: laughter alternates with

violent outbursts of weeping and anger with remorse or guilt
- May try to bottle feelings up in an effort to keep a 'stiff upper lip', until they explode to the surface in hysterical crying
- Sighs frequently as a result of feeling resentful and misunderstood
- Excitable, nervous, and twitchy
- Hypersensitive to noise, strong odours, pain and/or criticism

Head

- A tendency to headaches may date from an episode of stress or shock
- Exposure to strong smells or perfumes can trigger a headache
- Visual aura of zig-zags in front of the eyes with migraines makes it difficult to achieve and maintain visual focus
- Dizzy and unsteady with headaches due to a heavy, hot sensation in the head
- Sharp sensation as though a nail were sticking into the side, or back, of the head
- Headaches and migraines may be temporarily relieved by being sick and made worse by movement

Ears

- Tinnitus may come on, or be made more intense, as a result of mental and emotional stress

Respiratory (Nose and Throat)

- Headache with dry, unproductive head cold
- Sore throat and loss of voice develop after emotional upset or stress
- Sensation of obstruction or lump in the throat. This can be accompanied by tearfulness or holding tears back
- Sore throats feel more painful for swallowing saliva and drinking fluids and better for belching or eating

Digestive

- Lots of saliva in the mouth which has a bitter taste
- 'Repeating' of flavours from the stomach when belching or hiccuping
- Empty, hollow sensations in the stomach are temporarily relieved by eating
- Takes deep breaths in an effort to relieve unpleasant sinking feelings in the stomach
- Spasmodic, cramping pains in the belly associated with constipation
- Painless diarrhoea may be sparked off by emotional distress
- Striking and contradictory symptom of a soft stool being harder to pass than a firm one when suffering from constipation

Reproductive

- Periods are upset as a result of emotional trauma. This can result in irregular cycles, or menopausal symptoms, escalating
- Colicky, spasmodic period cramps that are relieved by rest, moving position or applying firm pressure
- During a period the flow may look dark and clotted; spasmodic cramps are at their most severe before clots are expelled
- Fast-moving mood swings after having a baby with lots of tears

Sleep

- Lots of twitching and jolting of muscles in light, fitful sleep
- Restless, disturbed sleep as a result of emotional trauma
- Whimpers and moans in sleep

Muscles and Joints

- Lots of tension and stiffness in the muscles: especially in the neck and lower back. Pains may extend from the back to the thighs
- Intermittent sciatica which is noticeably worse in cold weather, being so troublesome at night that it drives the sufferer out of bed in search of relief
- Pains are characteristically tingling and cramping

SYMPTOMS ARE TRIGGERED OR MADE WORSE BY:

- Trying to hide and suppress emotions
- Following emotional shock and trauma
- Grief (especially if feelings are not allowed their natural expression)
- Feeling fearful or anxious
- Too much sugar, alcohol and/or coffee (aggravates mood swings)
- Yawning
- Pressure applied to areas that aren't painful
- Becoming cold or chilled

SYMPTOMS ARE EASED BY:

- Warmth
- Being distracted
- Pressure applied to painful areas
- Eating

ipecac

Made from a homeopathic dilution of the ipecacuanha plant, this remedy can help ease: morning sickness that isn't relieved by severe vomiting; wheezy coughs and whooping cough.

Core Features

- Lingering nausea that is made much worse by the slightest movement
- Easy, frequent bleeding; nosebleeds may occur for very little reason
- Weary and wrung out

Emotional State

- Very touchy, grouchy and irritable in response to the slightest provocation
- Hypersensitive to noise; loud music in particular
- Anxious and fearful of death

- Impatient and dissatisfied
- Illness may be triggered by bottling up anger and irritability

Head
- Nauseating headache that feels worse for moving even slightly
- The whole skull feels bruised, or pains may lodge at the back of the head
- Exhausted and prostrated in waves when feeling ill
- Looks pale and drawn with headache and constant vomiting: even water is brought back up

Respiratory (Nose and Chest)
- Cold symptoms with lots of sneezing
- Nose feels either completely stuffed up, or streams with blood-streaked mucus
- Colds set off nosebleeds easily
- Lots of irritation and tickling in the throat sets off sudden coughing spasms
- Wheezing and breathlessness with coughing leads to gagging and retching that may cause actual vomiting
- Sensation of heaviness in the chest makes it difficult to lie down
- Rattling of mucus in the chest from congestion

Digestive
- Constant nausea that isn't eased by vomiting
- Nausea and vomiting are often triggered by overindulgence
- Colicky pains that centre around the area of the navel with nausea and vomiting
- Diarrhoea and distended belly with severe nausea and vomiting

Reproductive
- Flooding periods with feeling of faintness and sickness
- Period flow either oozes steadily, or may come in gushes; colour is likely to be bright red
- Heavy bleeding after childbirth

SYMPTOMS ARE TRIGGERED OR MADE WORSE BY:
- Extremes of warmth or cold temperatures
- Humidity
- Eating
- Light touch

SYMPTOMS ARE EASED BY:
- Firm pressure
- Resting with the eyes closed
- In the open air

kali bich

Prepared from a homeopathic dilution of Bichromate of potash this remedy can be useful in treating: bronchitis; catarrh; croup; German measles; headaches; post-nasal drip (mucus that drips down the back of the throat, often a complication of an established cold); sinusitis and wheezy coughs.

Core Features
- Weariness and exhaustion with marked chilliness
- Signature discharges (especially catarrhal secretions) are yellow, stringy and difficult to shift
- Pains are focused on one small spot or shift from place to place
- Conditions alternate from one organ system to another; e.g. digestive symptoms with rheumatic aches and pains
- Ulcers form rapidly and/or recurrently
- Symptoms respond very badly to becoming chilled

Emotional State
- Averse to the idea of making the slightest amount of mental or physical effort
- Anxious feelings centre in, or rise from the chest
- Meeting new people especially triggers anxiety
- Mentally exhausted and listless

- Problems with mental focus and concentration

Head
- Vomiting and nausea with dizziness
- Migraines with queasiness and nausea that are more severe at night
- Sinus headaches with tenderness and pain that lodge at the bridge of the nose
- One-sided headaches that affect the area above one eye
- Aching in the bones of the head and face

Eyes
- Burning and itching in dry, sensitive eyes
- Recurrent bouts of conjunctivitis with hot, inflamed eyeball
- General state of inflammation extends to the eyelids that look swollen and red at the margins

Respiratory (Throat, Nose and Chest)
- Irritating sensation as though a hair is resting on the tongue
- Lots of catarrh at the back of the throat that is stringy and difficult to cough up
- Painful, sore throat with an enlarged, puffy-looking uvula (the 'little tongue' that lies at the top of the throat)
- Lots of nasal mucus that burns the nostrils and upper lip
- Nasty smell in the nose from infected mucus
- Nose can also be dry and blocked with sticky, yellow mucus
- Breathless with harsh, croupy cough that causes gagging as a result of the effort to try and raise sticky mucus from the chest
- The effort of coughing up difficult mucus can trigger back pains
- If coughing bouts happen too soon after eating, this can lead to actual vomiting (especially in whooping cough)

Digestive

- Anxious, uneasy feeling in the stomach when feeling on edge
- Burping eases stomach upsets
- Colicky pains are relieved by firm pressure and warmth locally applied
- Abdominal bloating and distention comes on soon after eating

Sleep

- Poor, fitful sleep quality as a result of digestive upsets, coughing and/or breathlessness. This can lead to a tendency to wake around 2a.m.

Muscles and Joints

- Hip and knee pains are made more intense and distressing when moving around or standing
- Pain and soreness in the heels when walking
- Discomfort and aching in the shoulders that is more intense during the night
- Shooting pain from the buttock to calf muscle with sciatica that's more intense when walking

SYMPTOMS ARE TRIGGERED OR MADE WORSE BY:

- Chill, especially from exposure to dry, cold winds
- Uncovering
- During the winter months
- Bending or stooping forwards
- When waking from sleep
- When alone
- Getting too hot
- From 2–5a.m.

SYMPTOMS ARE EASED BY:

- Resting in bed
- Being warmly wrapped up
- During the summer months
- Firm pressure applied to painful areas
- During the daytime

kali carb

Made from a homeopathic dilution of Potassium carbonate, this remedy can be useful in treating: anaemia; back pain; bronchitis; catarrh; labour pains; pre-menstrual syndrome; sciatica; thrush; wheezy coughs and whooping cough.

Core Features

- Extreme sensitivity to cold with a tendency to be rapidly chilled
- General tendencies to develop fluid retention, puffiness and swelling (especially around the eye area)
- Odd symptom of burning pains in areas that feel locally cool to the touch
- Rapidly moving pains are eased temporarily by warmth that's locally applied
- Nature of pains tends to be characteristically stitching, or stabbing, in nature
- The right side of the body may be more affected than the left
- Weakness and lethargy can be related to underlying problems with anaemia

Emotional State

- Irritable and grouchy: at odds with everything and everyone
- Uptight and edgy; noticeably sensitive to noise or shocks of any kind
- Highly strung with problems in coping with stress
- Fearful and anxious with specific fears focused on being alone, or a fear of death
- Difficult to please

Head

- Burning pains in the cheekbones, above the eyes, and/or over the scalp
- Chronic pain and congestion triggers recurrent headaches
- Head pains are made more intense by exposure to cold air, and eased by firm pressure to the painful area and/or wrapping the head up warmly

Respiratory (Throat, Nose and Chest)

- Sharp pains and soreness in the throat with a feeling of swallowing over an obstruction or lump
- Nasty-tasting mucus and lumpy catarrh lingers on after the established stage of a cold and is difficult to shift
- Uncomfortably dry nasal passages with a marked tendency for the nose to block up in a warm room
- The nose looks very red and swollen
- Saliva gathers in the throat and mouth
- Hacking, dry chesty cough with puffy swelling of the upper eyelids
- Chilly feeling in the chest when wheezy
- Wheezy cough is eased by bending forwards and/or sitting up.
- Shooting, burning pains in the chest with a sense of pressure when breathing

Digestive

- Sinking feelings in the stomach are aggravated by eating
- Uncomfortable heavy feeling in the stomach after eating
- Swelling and bloating in the belly after eating with burping and flatulence
- Burning sensations with heartburn that's made more intense after cold drinks
- Colicky pains are soothed by locally-applied warmth in the form of a hot water bottle or warm compress
- Diarrhoea alternates with constipation accompanied by burning sensations in the rectum and anus. These are (unusually for this remedy) soothed by the local application of cool water

Reproductive
- Becomes noticeably chilly with cramping pains before the onset of a period
- Constipation is especially noticeable around the time of period pain
- Heavy flow with period pains that refuse to respond to usual conventional medical techniques (such as dilatation and curettage)
- Labour pains settle in the back during childbirth and/or back pain may be noticeable during pregnancy

Muscles and Joints
- Legs 'give out' without warning as a consequence of muscle weakness
- Pain and weakness in the back extends to the muscles of the thighs and is more intense pre-menstrually and when walking

SYMPTOMS ARE TRIGGERED OR MADE WORSE BY :
- Change in the weather
- Being chilled
- Light touch
- Becoming too hot
- Drinking coffee
- In the early morning

SYMPTOMS ARE EASED BY:
- Leaning or bending forward
- During the day
- Humid, warm weather

lachesis

Made from a homeopathic dilution of the surukuku snake venom, this remedy can be helpful in easing: hot flushes; migraines; mood swings (especially those that occur pre-menstrually or approaching menopause); mumps; night sweats; painful, clotted periods; pre-menstrual headaches; sleep problems; sore throats; swollen glands and varicose veins.

Core Features
- Poor circulation creates a signature mottled, purplish appearance to the skin. This is often associated with easy bruising or a tendency to varicose veins and piles
- Symptoms are characteristically left sided or move from the left to the right side of the body
- Symptoms are generally most intense when feeling hemmed in or constricted, becoming overheated or waking from sleep (a dread of going to bed or falling asleep can develop as a result)
- Sensitive to being touched around the throat and becoming overheated

Emotional State
- Fast mood changes alternate between euphoria and depression
- Very chatty with a tendency to talk non-stop and switch quickly from one subject to another
- Emotional problems are often linked to a poor sleep pattern
- Creative and imaginative by nature; works best late at night when ideas rush in and, as a result, feels energetic and full of vitality when it's time to be winding down and switching off
- Specific fear of dying in sleep makes it difficult to drift off
- Physical and mental exhaustion are not improved after a night's sleep

- Anxiety and depression are pronounced on waking and lift as the day goes on
- Moods shift sharply between bouts of confidence and low self-esteem

Head
- Headaches and migraines can be set off or aggravated by bright lights
- Headaches and/or migraines characteristically come on when waking from sleep and are more likely to be left-sided
- Headaches and migraines build in intensity as the date of the period comes closer and are eased as soon as the flow gets under way
- Upsetting dizziness is made more intense when closing the eyes

Respiratory (Throat, Nose and Chest)
- Pressure in the nose is relieved by the onset of a discharge such as a nosebleed or free flowing mucus
- Sneezing with blocked nose when waking from sleep
- Constricted feeling in the throat on waking
- All discomfort in the throat is made better for swallowing food and made worse for 'empty' swallowing (as in swallowing saliva)
- Strong dislike of any clothing that puts pressure on the throat such as a tight scarf or polo neck jumper

Digestive
- Wind and bloating are aggravated by tight, restrictive clothing and temporarily relieved by passing a stool
- Established problems with constipation and piles that bleed very easily

Reproductive
- Severe hot flushes, night sweats, and mood swings with the menopause
- Severe pre-menstrual symptoms,

such as ovarian pain (may be especially noticeable on the left side) and violent mood swings
• During a period the flow is dark in colour, clotted and very heavy

Flushes

• Hot flushes are made incredibly distressing when wearing anything that hugs the neck area
• Intolerance of warm, airless rooms and an obvious preference for cool, fresh atmospheres
• Rapidly shifts from feeling hot to cold

Sleep

• Nasty sensation of falling and jerking awake when drifting off to sleep
• Sleep problems often include feelings of panic, palpitations, suffocation, anxiety and actual panic attacks
• Bad dreams trigger feelings of disorientation and distress on waking

SYMPTOMS ARE TRIGGERED OR MADE WORSE BY:

• Sleep
• Heat
• Stuffy rooms
• During the night
• Being chilled
• Hot sunlight
• Alcohol
• Tight clothes
• From ovulation to the onset of a period

SYMPTOMS ARE EASED BY:

• Cold drinks
• Contact with fresh, cool air
• Once a discharge appears
• Moving around
• Eating solid food
• As the day goes on

ledum

Made from a homeopathic dilution of wild rosemary, this remedy can be helpful in easing any of the following conditions: bruises; black eyes; insect stings; joint pains; joint sprains; muscle strains; osteoarthritis and puncture wounds.

Core Features

• Signature pains are sharp and stabbing by nature
• They also tend to move about, especially from the lower parts of the body to the upper ones
• Tendency to swollen, taut injuries, often associated with puffiness and fluid retention
• Strange, characteristic symptom of painful area feeling stiff, numb and chilly, but relieved by cool bathing and/or applying cool compresses
• General sensation of aching, bruised pains through the whole body
• Hard, painful swelling with tearing pains
• Although feeling hot and swollen, affected joints don't appear red or inflamed

Emotional State

• Cross, bad tempered and withdrawn
• Low, depressed with lots of sighing in between bouts of crying

Muscles and Joints

• Hot, stiff joints that look swollen. They respond well temporarily to cool bathing and cool applications but are made noticeably worse for contact with warmth such as the heat of the bed
• Joint pains move upwards through the body
• Pain and stiffness in the lower back is aggravated by sitting still in one position for too long
• Joint pain and stiffness is associated with passing large amounts of pale coloured urine

Skin

• Itching and discomfort of the skin are aggravated by exposure to heat but feel instantly better for contact with cool air, and/or cool water
• Puncture wounds, bruises and black eyes feel cool to the touch

SYMPTOMS ARE TRIGGERED OR MADE WORSE BY :

• At night
• Warmth in any form
• Walking
• Alcohol
• Being well covered or wrapped up

SYMPTOMS ARE EASED BY:

• Cool compresses
• Uncovering and allowing for contact with cool air
• Rest
• Cool bathing

lycopodium

Made from a homeopathic dilution of club moss, this remedy can be useful in treating: anxiety; burn out; constipation; diarrhoea; digestive upsets; eczema; headaches; heartburn; indigestion; low libido; prostate problems; psoriasis; sore throats and wheezing.

Core Features

• Signature symptoms include all sort of digestive upsets, but especially including the production of excess wind in stomach and belly, plus a noticeable amount of distension and bloating accompanied by huge amounts of noisy rumbling and gurgling
• Symptoms get characteristically much worse, or come on, between

4 and 8p.m. They then lift and improve as the night goes on
• Symptoms move from the right to the left side of the body
• Low quality of physical stamina with a pronounced tendency to become exhausted after making a moderate amount of physical effort

Emotional State

• Although domineering and bossy on the surface, underneath feels insecure and anxious. This breaks through and surfaces as a specific fear of failing when speaking in public. Although terrified with lots of anxiety before the event, when it gets under way it generally goes very well
• Very sensitive to criticism and easily made irritable when feeling challenged. Flies off the handle when corrected
• Constantly preoccupied or worried about finances, with a fear of losing a grip on day-to-day affairs. This comes from a deep-seated anxiety and fear about losing control and confronting failure
• Tendency to lack of mental focus and concentration when over-tired and over-worked
• Hurries in speech and movement
• Appears detached and lacking in emotional responsiveness Intellectual abilities may have been nurtured at the expense of emotional spontaneity
• Dislikes feeling personal space is being invaded but also uncomfortable with being totally solitary. Ideal situation is being alone, with someone whose company can be called on when feeling the need

Head

• Dizziness is made more intense by eating, drinking or talking
• Headaches come on as a result of skipping or delaying meals with resulting plummeting blood sugar levels

• Headaches with severe crushing pains that are made more uncomfortable by exposure to warmth, or lying down. Pains are eased by gentle exercise in the open air

Eyes

• Tendency to recurrent or regular stye formation with pussy, sticky discharges
• Irritated, dry eyes and eyelids with swelling

Respiratory (Throat, Nose and Chest)

• Sore throats with a tendency to develop ulcers. Pains are temporarily soothed by warm drinks and made more uncomfortable for cold drinks
• Burning, constricted, choking feelings in the throat
• Lots of thick, yellowish-green mucus that collects at the back of the throat
• Recurrent problems with sinus congestion, discomfort and blocked nasal passages
• Headaches from frequent and severe coughing spasms
• Coughing bouts are triggered by inhaling deeply and/or swallowing saliva
• Shallow breathing when sleeping, or when involved in physical exertion
• Sense of rawness and pressure in the chest, which can feel more uncomfortable and intense after speaking

Digestive

• Digestive problems are most often triggered or linked to underlying issues with anxiety and stress, especially in the anticipatory phase
• Sensitivity and weakness of digestive organs. Starts a meal feeling hungry but quickly feels too full to finish what is on the plate. Then hunger sets in an hour or so after eating

• Incomplete, sour-tasting burps that leave a burning sensation in the gullet after they've come up
• Acidity and discomfort develop quickly after eating and are soothed temporarily by sipping warm drinks
• General digestive uneasiness is aggravated by pressure of a tight waist band pressing on the belly
• Heartburn and indigestion are established or frequent features as a result of excess acid production and/or accumulation of wind
• Alternation between constipation and diarrhoea means that achieving an easy, daily, smooth bowel movement is rare

Urination

• Strong-smelling, dark, cloudy-looking urine
• Frequent sensation of needing to urinate at night
• Aches and pains in the loin area (at the sides of the body) are severe before passing water, and eased afterwards
• Males who suffer from prostate enlargement find that flow of urine is slow to start

Reproductive

• Low libido when stressed, with males experiencing some degree of erectile dysfunction with a tendency to premature ejaculation
• Noticeable pre-menstrual syndrome symptoms with headaches, depression and lots of abdominal distention and bloating
• Severe cramps with period pains that extend from the lower back to the front of the thighs. Cramping pains are temporarily eased by drawing knees up into the abdomen
• Marked itching in the vagina with or without a smelly, copious discharge
• Odd sensation as though wind were moving through the vagina
• Periods become flooding, clotted and dark as the menopause gets closer

Flushes and Fever

- Sudden, severe hot flushes as a result of emotional stress, strain and anxiety. One the flush is retreating it leaves an unpleasant feeling of cold clamminess
- Frequency and severity of flushes are made more intense by feeling hemmed in, wearing tight, restrictive clothing, or being in demanding company
- Although feeling noticeably chilly, there is a noticeable aversion to getting too hot, or being in poorly ventilated surroundings

Skin

- The scalp is intensely itchy and scaly with an obvious tendency to develop dandruff. The hair may become dry, brittle and easily broken as well as the nails
- Skin is generally dry and irritated with burning, frequently burning and feeling itchy
- Irritation becomes more noticeable, severe and problematic when becoming hot in bed, and relieved by contact with comfortably cool air or applying cool compresses

SYMPTOMS ARE TRIGGERED OR MADE WORSE BY:

- First thing in the morning
- In the mid to late afternoon and early evening
- On waking from sleep
- Warm, stuffy, overheated rooms
- Draughts of very cold air
- Tight restrictive clothes
- Heavy bed covers
- Excessive stress loads that overtire

SYMPTOMS ARE EASED BY:

- Moderate, comfortable levels of warmth
- Uncovering when too hot
- Wearing loose, comfortable clothes
- Gentle exercise in the fresh air

mercuris

Prepared from a homeopathic dilution of quicksilver, this remedy can be useful in treating: abscesses; boils; breast tenderness; catarrh; chickenpox; earache; flu; mouth ulcers; mumps; sinus congestion; sore throat; tonsillitis and swollen glands.

Core Features

- All symptoms (emotional and physical) are much more unpleasant and distressing at night
- Extreme weariness and lethargy may be linked to post-viral problems or anaemia
- Extreme temperatures result in restlessness, uneasiness and a general sense of discomfort
- Recurrent or persistent inflammation, pain and swelling in the glands of the neck, armpits and groin
- Offensive smell of discharges such as saliva, mucus and/or sweat
- An underlying tendency to fluid retention leads to puffiness and swelling of the fingers, ankles, face or feet

Emotional State

- Anxious, restless and fearful for no obvious cause: moves about constantly from one position to another
- Emotional distress is noticeably more intense during the night
- Anxiety leads to panic attacks with a feeling of wanting to run away and escape
- Either very flustered and hyper, or indifferent, withdrawn and apathetic
- Mild to moderate depression leads to poor memory and unrealistic assessment of rate at which time is passing

Ears

- Earache is especially distressing and distracting at night
- Sharp pains in the ears with thick, offensive-smelling discharge

Respiratory (Throat, Nose and Chest)

- Difficult to swallow because of the amount of soreness and dryness in the throat but there's an annoying tendency to need to keep doing it, due to an excessive amount of saliva produced by the salivary glands in the mouth
- Large, painful, sensitive ulcers in the mouth and throat
- Recurrent or persistently swollen glands
- Soreness and rawness of the nostrils with production of thick, offensive mucus
- Episodes of coughing with associated nausea are worse at night, when lying on the right side or when lying down

Sleep

- Because of problems drifting off into a sound, refreshing sleep at night there's a lot of drowsiness during the day
- Awful restlessness at night from a strong sense of physical uneasiness. This is made worse by a tendency to heavy, offensive-smelling night sweats
- Wakes frequently during the night with palpitations, anxious feelings and drenching sweats

Digestive

- Nasty, sweetish, metallic taste in the mouth with a noticeably increased amount of salvia being produced. This is made even worse and more intense when sensations of nausea are around
- Tongue looks and feels enlarged to the point of taking the imprint of the teeth
- Stomach upsets are triggered or made worse by eating too many sugary foods
- Stomach cramps and diarrhoea are made more severe and

uncomfortable when stooping forward or bending
• Watery, burning diarrhoea gets progressively worse at night

Flushes and Fever
• Hot flushes alternate with feeling chilled and clammy
• The body remains chilled while hot flushes affect the head and face
• Very thirsty with drenching perspiration

Skin
• Last stage of boil formation with greenish-yellow thick pus

Muscles and Joints
• Low, burning back pains that radiate to the thighs. The neck is also painful and stiff from muscle tension
• Awful muscular restlessness and aching in the arms and legs that get progressively more intense as the night goes on
• Restless legs in an effort to try to get into a comfortable position in bed at night
• Cramping pains and stiffness in the joints of the fingers and hands

SYMPTOMS ARE TRIGGERED OR MADE WORSE BY :
• Getting warm in bed
• During the evening and the night
• Extreme temperatures from very hot to very cold
• Becoming chilled by draughts of cold air
• Eating
• When perspiring
• Being touched
• Lying on the right hand side

SYMPTOMS ARE EASED BY:
• Finding a comfortable position to rest in
• Moderate, consistent temperatures

natrum mur
Made from a homeopathic dilution of common salt, this remedy can help treat: allergic rhinitis; catarrh; cold sores; constipation; cracked, dry chapped skin; eczema; hay fever; headaches; migraines; morning sickness; pre-menstrual syndrome; prickly heat; post-natal depression and thrush.

Core Features
• Think of this remedy for situations where symptoms are associated with marked shifts in hormone levels. Suitable candidates include mood swings around a menstrual bleed, pre-menstrual or menopausal headaches or migraines, and fluid retention
• Symptoms of illness often develop after emotions have been suppressed associated with bereavement, grief and relationship break up
• An underlying tendency to allergic responses such as hives, prickly heat, allergic rhinitis, and stress-related skin reactions and hay fever
• Warmth and exposure to direct sunshine aggravate or trigger headaches, rashes and hot flushes
• Dryness and sensitivity of the skin and mucus membranes
• Exhaustion and weariness that are especially marked in the morning

Emotional State
• Very withdrawn and introverted with the classic British 'stiff upper lip' to emotional uptightness
• Crying doesn't provide any release from distress because it leads to feeling humiliated and embarrassed: especially if this happens in public
• Although feeling really unhappy and low, displays of sympathy and emotion just make everything worse. This is often linked to fear of bursting into tears
• Moods alternate between excitability, sadness and euphoria
• Although disliking lots of attention and fuss, feels easily lonely and neglected if feeling overlooked
• Cries in private when upset and distressed and tends to bottle up other feelings such as anger and resentment
• Emotional symptoms tend to be at their most intense at times of major hormonal shifts such as puberty, pregnancy, and approaching and during menopause

Head
• Having meals delayed can trigger headaches, as well as being more likely to come on before, during or after a period. This remedy can also be indicated for the treatment of menopausal migraines
• The pain of headaches feels more intense for moving around and is relieved by lying down and sleeping
• Migraine headaches with tingling, numb sensations in the lips, nose and tongue, with visual disturbance. This takes the form of a zig-zag pattern before the eyes

Eyes
• Hayfever with very itchy, sensitive, swollen eyes
• Gritty, dry eyes that water very quickly when out in cold winds

Respiratory (Throat, Nose and Chest)
• Recurrent colds, allergic rhinitis or hayfever that starts off with lots of bouts of repeated sneezing
• Tendency to cold sores that break out around the nose and mouth. Common triggers include colds, exposure to strong sunlight, emotional stress and strain or being run down
• The nose may either run like a

tap with lots of watery, clear mucus coming away, or it can be jelliy-like. During a cold or hayfever, symptoms can alternate between the two states
• Lips and mouth show strong tendencies for the skin to be dry, sensitive and cracked. This can affect the middle of the bottom lip or the corners of the mouth especially
• The throat feels dry and tickly
• Coughing spasms can be triggered by an irritating, persistent tickle coming from the throat
• The lungs may feel tight

Digestive
• Discomfort and uneasiness in the stomach with a tendency for 'repeating' of flavours of food eaten a while ago
• Sinking feeling in the stomach with queasiness
• Noticeable craving for salty foods: this may be especially strong around the time of a period. Or alternatively, a strong aversion to salty things can also suggest this remedy is well indicated
• Colicky pains and nausea are temporarily eased by passing wind
• Heavy, sluggish sensation in the stomach with a tendency to stubborn constipation
• Strains to pass dry, hard stools

Urination
• Finds it difficult to pass water when others can hear: takes a long time for the flow to get started
• Passes large amounts of pale-coloured urine
• Stress incontinence with dribbling of urine when sneezing, coughing, laughing or exercising

Reproductive
• Lack of tone of pelvic organs with a tendency for the womb and/or bladder to prolapse. This is most likely to happen in mid life,

but can happen at an earlier age after pregnancies that have occurred close together
• A tendency to low back pain may be associated with a prolapse Pains are eased by applying firm pressure to the hollow of the back when lying or sitting
• Established dryness of the vagina can trigger an aversion to intercourse due to the smarting, sensitive sensations that happen during and/or afterwards
• Severe nausea and morning sickness in pregnancy with vomiting of watery, frothy phlegm
• Periods may be slow to start, early, heavy or associated with a scanty flow
• Noticeable fluid retention pre-menstrually with associated breast tenderness and swelling with discomfort around the waist

Sleep
• Problems surface when initially falling asleep, or once fully asleep wakes frequently during the night thinking of distressing thoughts
• Night sweats in the second half of the night

Flushes and Fever
• Feels hot and bothered with palpitations and flushes
• Flushes rise quickly and abruptly to the head and chest, but the lower half of the body stays cool

Skin
• Skin is very dry and sensitive with a marked tendency to crack easily. This is most pronounced during the winter months
• Very itchy, blotchy, irritated skin from exposure to strong sunlight and/or extremely hot conditions
• Sensitive skin is aggravated by contact with heat in any form, and noticeably soothed by cool bathing and uncovering to expose the skin to cool air

SYMPTOMS ARE TRIGGERED OR MADE WORSE BY:
• Emotional trauma or stress
• Being hugged or shown lots of sympathy
• Getting over-excited
• After a good cry
• Waking from sleep
• Extreme temperatures
• Getting too hot
• Lack of fresh air
• Too much physical effort
• During or at the end of a period

SYMPTOMS ARE EASED BY:
• Being left in peaceful, quiet surroundings
• Exposure to cool air
• Skipping meals
• Gentle exercise that doesn't cause exhaustion to set in
• Sea air (although this can also sometimes aggravate symptoms)
• Tight, restricting clothing

nux vomica
Made from a homeopathic dilution using the dried seeds of the Strychnos nux vomica plant. Known for its primary action as a de-toxing remedy, Nux vomica can be helpful in treating: anxiety; burn out; colic; constipation; cystitis; digestive upsets related to overindulgence and high stress levels; haemorrhoids; hangover headaches; head colds; labour pains; muscle tension; painful periods; poor sleep pattern and sleep quality; tension headaches and stress-related migraines.

Core Features
• One of the primary remedies to consider when a hangover develops, or when feeling generally 'toxic' and run down as a result of eating and/or drinking unwisely, or relying too much on painkillers or coffee and/or alcohol in order to

keep the pace
• This remedy can also be useful if side-effects are left after a course of conventional medication. Symptoms that can respond especially positively include constipation or rebound headaches that follow use of painkillers, or stomach upsets that are associated with using anti-inflammatories
• Symptoms are commonly associated with an overly-stressful lifestyle that isn't managed well by adequate stress-reduction measures. Instead, negative patterns may emerge in response to the stress load that may include over-reliance on sleeping tablets, painkillers, coffee, alcohol, cigarettes and/or junk foods that are high in sugar and chemical additives
• Oversensitivity on physical, mental and emotional levels leads to a tendency to be 'short-fused' and very irritable in response to minimum provocation. Physical oversensitivity takes the form of extreme sensitivity to noise, disturbance and cold, draughty conditions
• All symptoms are more intense and distressing on first waking in the morning, improving steadily as the day goes on
• Signature pains are tight, cramping, constrictive and spasmodic in nature

Emotional State

• Hypersensitivity with severe and/or recurrent problems with poor sleep pattern which is characteristically light and fitful
• Underlying currents of irritability, frustration and discontent that surface quickly in response to very minor triggers
• Sensitive to criticism with an aversion to consolation and sympathy
• Picks quarrels when feeling out of sorts and ill and feels generally better for an explosive outburst

• Tense, uptight and unable to switch off after work. This situation is unwittingly made more severe by the negative coping strategies mentioned above
• Anxious and tense about work, health, and financial security

Head

• Classic tension headaches that extend from tightness at the back of the head. Pain and discomfort are made more intense by exposure to cold draughts and chilly conditions in general, while warmth, peace and quiet and firm pressure all help ease the pain
• Sick headaches associated with constipation, nausea and total lack of interest in eating anything
• Hangover headaches with disorientation, dizziness, pain that lodges at the back of the head, queasy stomach, and hypersensitivity to noise, strong smells, and generally being disturbed
• Tense, tight feelings with headaches that are eased after achieving a sound sleep
• Muzzy headedness with headaches

Respiratory (Throat, Nose and Chest)

• Head cold symptoms are generally more unpleasant and distressing in a warm room and temporarily eased by taking a gentle stroll in the open air
• Colds trigger an unpleasant irritation and itching in the ears
• Shooting pains travel to the ears between swallowing
• Lots of sneezing with raw feeling in the throat
• The nose is hypersensitive to strong smells with the nasal passages being alternately stuffed up and dry, or running like a tap
• Coughing bouts are soothed by warm drinks and made more intense by exposure to cold draughts of air
• Headaches come on as a result of coughing spasms

• Irritating, tickly dry cough that is more severe at night

Digestive

• Digestive uneasiness and upsets are triggered or made more severe by high stress levels, too much tea, coffee, alcohol, eating badly (this can either involve relying on junk foods or lots of eating out), and smoking too much
• Eating makes indigestion, colicky pains and wind worse, while warmth and rest are soothing
• Persistent sick feeling with awful difficulty in vomiting. This is due to something called reverse persistalsis, where food seems determined to stay in the stomach rather than travelling freely and easily upwards in order to be expelled. This process can also affect the bowel, making it very difficult indeed to pass a complete stool. As a result, there can be a troublesome feeling of incompleteness after passing a stool
• Lots of flushing after eating with unpleasant feelings of sleepiness and drowsiness
• Stress and anxiety make the stomach feel uneasy, sick and heavy: all of these are made more intense after eating

Urination

• Severe pain and difficulty passing water, with burning pains especially affecting the right side of the body
• Pain and distress in the bladder is especially severe at night. There may be itching sensations when passing water

Reproductive

• Noticeable pre-menstrual syndrome symptoms, with marked emotional short-fuse, bursts of temper and irritability
• Becomes faint and chilly with period pains
• Dry retching in labour, with difficulty in raising stomach

contents. This is likely to be accompanied by outbursts of temper, irritability and aggression

Sleep

- Problems mentally and physically switching off, and so may develop a habit of relying on alcohol or sleeping pills in order to get off to sleep
- Poor quality, light, fitful easily-broken sleep for most of the night and early morning but falls into a deep sleep when it's time to get up
- Feels revived and refreshed for taking a nap during the day
- Poor quality sleep is disturbed by bad dreams

Muscles and Joints

- Joints and muscles feel stiff and painful to move when first getting up in the morning
- Joints and muscles feel weak and generally react negatively to exposure to chilled, cold conditions
- Lots of muscle cramps that are especially noticeable at night. These have a particular tendency to lodge in the calf muscles

SYMPTOMS ARE TRIGGERED OR MADE WORSE BY:

- Lack of sound, refreshing sleep
- First thing in the morning
- After eating
- Too many cigarettes
- Habitual use of alcohol, coffee and painkillers to cope with stress
- Exposure to strong smells
- Too much mental and emotional pressure and strain
- Constipation
- Noisy, disturbing surroundings

SYMPTOMS ARE EASED BY:

- Warm, peaceful surroundings
- Sound, refreshing sleep
- As the day goes on
- Achieving a complete bowel movement

phosphorus

Made from a homeopathic dilution of yellow phosphorus, this remedy is helpful in treating: anaemia; anxiety; baby blues; catarrh; coughs; croup; diarrhoea; food poisoning; hot flushes; nosebleeds; sinusitis; sore throats; swollen glands; tonsilitis and vomiting.

Core Features

- Underlying state of free-floating anxiety is present with many complaints. This sort of anxiety can attach itself to anything that presents itself as a potential source of worry
- Exhaustion is a central part of feeling ill, leading to a general feeling of being lacking in stamina. This may, or may not, be linked to underlying tendencies to anaemia
- Burning sensations can pop up anywhere in the body, with poor circulation leading to alternating flushes of heat, and bouts of chilliness
- Erratic energy levels with short bursts of energy alternating with apathy, lethargy and feelings of being 'burnt out'
- Swelling and puffiness of the fingers, hands, eyelids and feet.
- Mucus and catarrhal discharges are yellow tinged and/or blood-streaked

Emotional State

- Hypersensitive and reactive to a wide range of stimuli. These can include light, colour, music, touch and perfume
- Highly sympathetic with an almost psychic streak that can pick up on general atmospheres and people's specific moods. This can be a blessing in making someone highly sensitive but a curse in making it difficult to set down and maintain psychological boundaries

- Craving for physical affection and reassurance: responds incredibly well to reassurance and comfort
- Quickly mentally, emotionally and physically drained
- Lots of fears and worries are linked to having a vivid, impressionable mind and imagination. Specific fears include being alone, illness, thunderstorms, and spiders
- Although very vivacious, likeable and outgoing, becomes apathetic, irritable and withdrawn when exhausted and drained. This can lead to being very emotional with bouts of weepiness
- Feeling neglected leads to problems with anxiety and low mood. Perks up quickly in response to displays of care, attention and sympathy

Head

- Headache and nausea are a consequence of feeling weak and wobbly. This may be triggered by changes in atmospheric pressure (such as before a thunderstorm) and/or going too long without eating or drinking
- Flushed, burning face with a headache. Pains and discomfort are made more intense by being in warm stuffy rooms and lying down, while they are relieved by eating a little light food and contact with cool, fresh air
- Disorientation and wooziness when getting up too quickly from a stooping, or sitting position. This can also be triggered by turning the head swiftly or bending forward

Respiratory (Throat, Nose and Chest)

- Painless hoarseness or complete loss of voice
- Sore throat with noticeable sensitivity to being touched and inhaling cold air
- Colds quickly travel to the throat and chest with associated swelling and inflammation of the glands of the neck

• Stuffed up nasal passages make it very difficult to breathe freely and easily at night
• Coughs in an effort to clear the throat. The cough is likely to be dry, tickly and irritating and made more severe by moving from one temperature to another, or when lying down flat
• The chest and coughing spasms are eased by sitting propped up in bed and by stable, warm temperatures

Digestive

• Stuffy, overheated rooms make nausea and vomiting more intense and distressing
• Burning pains in the stomach with weak, queasy feelings that are temporarily soothed by taking drinks of cold water. Once this gets warmed up by the stomach it is vomited back up again
• Persistent nausea with burning fullness in the stomach
• Burping feels unpleasant and distressing, partly due to the unpleasant taste that comes into the throat with each belch
• Warm food and drinks are quickly vomited back up again
• Profuse diarrhoea without cramps can be passed involuntarily

Urination

• Burning sensations with a constant urge to pass small amounts of concentrated urine
• Blood-tinged discoloured urine that can have an oily or greasy-looking surface to it
• Increased thirst with frequent passing of pale coloured urine. If this symptom is established and persistent, a doctor should be consulted in order to do a blood test to rule out irregularities with blood sugar levels

Reproductive

• Pre-menstrual syndrome with lots of weepiness and feeling low and depressed
• Periods are long-lasting and heavy. They may tend towards flooding leading up to menopause
• Peri menopausal problems include anxiety (often combined with, or preceding, hot flushes), palpitations and clotted, bright red, gushing periods

Flushes and Fever

• Feelings of anxiety and foreboding precede a hot flush
• Sudden variations in blood flow trigger bouts of chilliness that alternate with sporadic flushes of heat
• Although feeling as though burning up, the hands and feet may feel icy cold

Muscles and Joints

• Sore, painful spine and hip joints that are highly sensitive to the slightest touch
• Burning pains in the spine when in bed at night, while the legs and knees feel icy cold
• Burning, tingling, itching, numb sensations affect the spine, back, arms and fingers

SYMPTOMS ARE TRIGGERED OR MADE WORSE BY:

• Lots of excitement
• When alone
• In the dark
• Thunderstorms
• Lying on the left side
• Damp, cold conditions
• Crowded surroundings
• Heights

SYMPTOMS ARE EASED BY:

• Massage
• Reassurance
• Physical displays of affection and sympathy
• Sound sleep
• Warmth (with the exception of stomach problems)
• Eating small amounts often

pulsatilla

Made from a homeopathic dilution of the wind-flower or meadow anemone, this remedy is helpful in any of the following conditions: arthritis; catarrh; chickenpox; chilblains; coughs; depression and baby blues; breast tenderness; digestive upsets such as indigestion and overindulgence; earache; established stage of colds and/or flu; grief; hayfever; headaches (especially pre-menstrual ones); heartburn in pregnancy; hot flushes; irregular periods; labour pains; night sweats; measles; morning sickness; mumps; painful periods; pre-menstrual syndrome; sinusitis; stress incontinence; swollen glands; styes; teething; thrush and varicose veins.

Core Features

• Think of this remedy where problems develop slowly and insidiously over the space of a few days. A typical situation would include the established stage of a cold, where mucus discharges have become thick and yellowish-green in colour. As a result, Pulsatilla is not a likely candidate for treating the initial stage of illness but far more often indicated in a later stage. A good example would include Measles once the rash has come out fully, or where catarrhal symptoms have become persistent and/or severe
• Symptoms by their nature are shifting, variable and changeable. The instability has an emotional as well as a physical dimension, with mood swings accompanying changeable physical symptoms
• Problems are linked to the effects of shifting hormone levels, with the result that this remedy is frequently indicated for symptoms arising at puberty, during and/or

following pregnancy and leading up to menopause
• All symptoms are relieved by gentle movement in the fresh air which has a beneficial effect in toning up a sluggish circulation. They are aggravated and made more intense when lying down or resting
• Signature unusual symptoms include chilliness with aggravation from, and aversion to, contact with warmth, but relief from cool in any form and dry mouth without thirst
• Discharges are characteristically bland, thick, and yellowish-green in colour
• Symptoms are typically limited to, or more intense on, the right side of the body

Emotional State
• Unstable, shifting, quickly changing moods that move from tearfulness to irritability, depression, anxiety, and happiness
• Emotional insecurity and changes of mood are especially severe pre-menstrually or when pregnant
• Emotional distress is significantly eased and lifted by being given consolation, sympathy and lots of affection
• Poor self-esteem and general lack of self-confidence leads to indecision and inability to stick to a decision
• When anxious and depressed there is a great need for reassurance, consolation and emotional support
• When upset feels much better after a good cry in sympathetic company
• Fearful and anxious in crowds, open spaces, when alone, and very fearful of losing their reason
• Timid, shy and in need of an awful lot of attention and encouragement
• Children become clingy, weepy and very demanding when feeling ill

Head
• Headaches with upset stomach from eating too many rich fatty foods, especially if combined with sitting in an overly-stuffy, overheated room
• Headaches come on, or get more severe, after eating. They may also have a tendency to get worse as the evening comes on
• Dizziness when getting up after lying down, or when walking out of doors
• Headaches are eased by applying firm pressure and/or cool flannels to the painful area, or generally eased by talking a gentle stroll in the fresh, cool open air

Eyes
• Itchy eyes with yellow, thick discharge that sticks the eyelids together in a yellow crust during sleep
• Recurrent styes may affect the lower lid
• Constant desire to rub the eyes as a result of irritation, burning and itching

Ears
• Ear pains are brought on by exposure to chill and draughts of cold air
• Earaches are accompanied by thick, yellow-coloured discharge. There's also likely to be muffled, deaf feeling with congestion and pain
• Heat and inflammation of the outer part of the ear

Respiratory (Throat, Nose and Chest)
• Sore, dry throat with no thirst.
• Swollen, sore nose with a cold that leads to associated loss of taste and smell
• Blocked nostrils that alternate from one side to another. The sensation is eased by contact with fresh air and made more distressing in warm stuffy rooms
• Catarrh is lingering, thick, bland

and yellowish-green in colour
• Tickly, dry cough during the night that alternates with a loose, productive cough once up and about in the morning
• Congested feeling in the chest on lying down that is eased by sitting up and/or moving around
• Phlegm that's raised is thick and yellowish-green in colour

Digestive
• Thick-coated surface to the tongue with stomach upsets. This may be white or yellow tinged
• Nasty taste in dry mouth without any marked increase in thirst
• Burning indigestion is made more uncomfortable by taking warm food or drinks and soothed by cool food and drinks
• Burps bring up flavour of food eaten previously
• Craving for indigestible foods such as cheese, pork, butter and cream
• Nausea and vomiting can be triggered by emotional stress, upset or excitement
• Diarrhoea can be set off by eating too much fruit and/or ice cream. It can begin, or be more intense at night
• Itchy, painful haemorrhoids that may protrude. These are made more severe and uncomfortable by becoming hot and are soothed by contact with cool

Urination
• Recurrent or persistent cystitis with burning, smarting sensations that are aggravated by becoming hot and bothered and eased by cool locally applied
• Pains and soreness continue even after passing water
• Discomfort in the bladder is made more uncomfortable when lying on the back in bed
• Involuntary leaking of urine when coughing, sneezing, lying down or walking

Flushes and Fever
• Although generally chilly, there's a strong aversion to becoming overheated in stuffy rooms
• Alternating hot and cold flushes with a sense of being very uncomfortable when being wrapped up too warmly
• Feels most comfortable when near an open window with gives ready access to cool, fresh air

Sleep
• Feels tired, sleepy and drowsy on going to bed but is disturbed by feeling too hot and sweaty during the night
• Restless and unable to get comfortable during the night. Throws off the covers, gets chilled, and pulls them back up again
• Sleeps with arms extended above the head and feet pushed out of the covers in search of a cool spot

Reproductive
• Irregular or late periods
• Changeable, clotted flow that may be very heavy and then become scanty
• Severe symptoms of Pre-menstrual syndrome with sensitive, enlarged breasts and mood swings
• Underlying tendencies to develop thrush with lots of violent itching and irritation. Discharge is thick and whitish-yellow in appearance
• Menopausal symptoms include abrupt onset of hot flushes with lack of tolerance of heat, low back pain, stress incontinence, and flooding, erratic periods
• All day morning sickness gets progressively worse as the evening and night come on
• Labour pains that are changeable, feeble, or slow to start may call for this remedy

Muscles and Joints
• Flitting changeable pains that shift rapidly from one area of the body to another
• Sensation of heavy legs during the day that ache in bed at night
• Immobility and stiffness of the muscle and joints that feel most severe on first moving about after rest and becoming hot, and are made more comfortable for gentle movement, contact with cool air and firm pressure

SYMPTOMS ARE TRIGGERED OR MADE WORSE BY :
• Overheated stuffy rooms
• Lack of contact with fresh air
• Being wrapped up too snuggly
• Humid conditions
• Resting
• Lying down
• In the evening and at night
• During or following pregnancy
• Approaching and moving through menopause

SYMPTOMS ARE EASED BY:
• Lots of sympathy and affection
• Having a good cry
• Contact with cool, fresh air
• Cool bathing
• Gentle exercise
• Firm pressure to a painful part

rhus tox
Made from a homeopathic dilution of poison ivy, this remedy can be helpful in treating: allergic rashes; arthritic pain; chicken pox; chilblains; cold sores; eczema; flu; measles; mild to moderate depression; mumps; poor, disturbed sleep pattern; sciatica; strains and sprains and swollen glands.

Core Features
• Think of this as the 'rusty hinge' remedy: with pains, stiffness and discomfort being noticeably more intense on first moving after rest, and easing once limbered up (provided moving around isn't continued to the point of overdoing it)
• Pain and stiffness come on after exposure to cold, damp weather
• Symptoms generally respond well to warm bathing
• Discomfort and distress are typically more intense during the night when resting in bed. This applies to emotional and physical symptoms
• Most symptoms are associated with extreme restlessness
• This is one of the main homeopathic remedies to consider for skin rashes that are blistery and intensely itchy, or tingly and itchy (as in the case of cold sores)

Emotional State
• Extreme mental and emotional restlessness that is especially distressing during the night
• Apathetic, withdrawn and depressed: seems to be lacking interest in everything
• Anxiety and fear with sadness and weepiness over things that normally wouldn't cause an upset. Bursts into floods of tears for no obvious reason
• Depression and restless anxiety are at their most severe when in bed at night
• Irritable and jittery with anxieties about financial affairs, business and domestic pressures, or there may be just a general, pervasive fear about the future
• Broods on unsettling and distressing episodes from the past, especially during the night when there's little around to provide a distraction

Head
• Headaches come on as a result of frustration, anger or getting cold and damp
• Migraine headaches are eased by walking in the cool, open air
• Severe headaches are soothed by warmth and when bending the head backwards

Respiratory (Throat, Nose and Chest)

- Sneezing with frequent nosebleeds on waking
- Heat, swelling and inflammation of the nose with burning pain when the sensitive part is touched
- Painful, dry cracked lips with underlying tendency to develop cold sores
- Hoarseness and loss of voice that improves the more the voice is used
- Dry, sore throat with bruised pain when speaking and shooting pain on swallowing
- Raw feeling in chest with nasty, bloody or salty taste in the mouth
- Severe headache from coughing bouts
- Tickly, dry cough that's brought on by exposure to the least draught of cold, damp air

Digestive

- Sensitive, sore, coated tongue with red triangular tip
- Severe, colicky stomach pains are eased by moving around and bending double
- Nausea is more intense when lying down
- Painless, severe diarrhoea in the mornings

Flushes and Fever

- High temperature with trembling and sweating that's made worse for taking hot drinks
- Unquenchable thirst for cold drinks, especially during the night
- Restless and mutters in disturbed, fitful sleep

Sleep

- Constantly moves about the bed in an effort to find a comfortable spot
- Exhausted and depressed on waking from an unrestful, unrefreshing sleep with disturbed dreams

Skin

- Constant itchiness and irritation of the skin at night in bed, with a nagging need to scratch
- Blistery, puffy skin eruptions with intolerable itching and burning sensations

Muscles and Joints

- Aches and pains are brought on, or made worse by exposure to cold, damp, chilled conditions
- Awful, upsetting restlessness with joint pains that triggers constant movement in an effort to find a position that feels comfortable
- Aches and pains come on after physically over-doing it
- Severely painful, stiff swollen joints that are made more painful by rest, on initial movement and any physical activity that continues at an excessively demanding level for too long
- Painful, stiff neck that is worse in the morning on first moving around after a night's rest

SYMPTOMS ARE TRIGGERED OR MADE WORSE BY:

- Cold, damp, chilly weather
- Resting
- Too much physical effort
- When in bed
- Standing
- Initial movement after being still
- During the night
- Scratching

SYMPTOMS ARE EASED BY:

- Ongoing gentle movement that doesn't get to the point of exhaustion
- Warmth
- Warm bathing
- Warm compresses
- Wrapping up well

ruta

Made from a homeopathic dilution of the plant commonly-called rue. It can be helpful in treating: bruising; damaged Achilles tendon; eye strain; sciatica and tendonitis.

Core Features

- Aching pains in the joints and bones that are often a result of injury to the periosteum (the sheath that covers the bones, allowing for the attachment of tendons). Pains of this nature continue long after the date of initial injury and after the superficial bruising has healed
- Marked restlessness and difficulty in keeping still for any lengthy period of time
- Generally chilly, with a feeling of wanting to be kept as warm as possible
- Sleepy during the day with an inability to sleep soundly at night. This is partly due to a distracting urge to stretch the limbs
- Feels weary and exhausted with joint pains

Emotional State

- Depressed, weepy and/or irritable with joint pains
- Anxiety and restlessness that are especially noticeable in the evening

Eyes

- Eye strain and pain in the eyes that sets in after reading or doing fine work of any kind
- Burning, hot eyes with possible blurred vision that is more noticeable in the evening
- The eyes smart and water after being rubbed

Muscles and Joints

- Pains have an affinity for the knuckles, wrists, knees and/or ankles
- Weakness in the joints that is

most severe when going up or down steps or rising from a sitting position
• Bruised pains in the thighs make walking difficult
• Restless legs: moves them constantly in an effort to get into a comfortable position
• Bruised pain and discomfort in the spine and lower back that's made worse when sitting down and eased by lying on the back

SYMPTOMS ARE TRIGGERED OR MADE WORSE BY:

• Touch
• Resting
• Stooping
• Lying on the painful area
• Walking in the fresh air

SYMPTOMS ARE EASED BY:

• Warmth
• Moving around gently indoors

sepia

Made from a homeoeopathic dilution of cuttlefish ink, this remedy can be helpful in easing: baby blues; back pain; burn out; a flagging libido; headaches and migraines; hot flushes and night sweats; irregular periods; mild to moderate depression; morning sickness; painful periods; pre-menstrual syndrome; prolapse; thrush; stress incontinence and varicose veins.

Core Features

• Mental, emotional and physical exhaustion, weariness and flatness
• Pervading sense of lack of motivation and indifference are linked to energy levels that feel down to zero
• A general sense of sagging or drooping is present on several levels. There may also be a persistent sense of a lump or ball

anywhere in the body
• Poor circulation leads to an underlying tendency to unstable body temperature, varicose veins, and haemorrhoids
• Nausea and dizziness are typically caused by unstable blood sugar levels, and are aggravated by going for long periods of time without food. These problems can be typically much more intense in pregnancy and pre-menstrually
• Although there is such as sense of being drained and exhausted, all mental, emotional and physical symptoms are perked up by taking some vigorous exercise
• Often needed for feelings of depression that occur leading up to, and during the menopause, following childbirth and linked to pre-menstrual problems, if other symptoms agree

Emotional State

• Black depression with extreme mood swings and irritability
• Although feeling so weepy, little or no relief occurs after having a good cry
• Emotionally volatile, impatient and irritable with family members, especially when feelings swamped by domestic or emotional demands and responsibilities
• Although full of energy and very capable of meeting day-to-day tasks when feeling well, once ill health starts to get a grip strong feelings of being unable to cope develop
• When feeling burdened by responsibilities, feelings of anxiety and agitation take hold. Screams and shouts in frustration, or just wants to run away and hide from demand
• Absolutely lacking in energy, vitality and drive: feels totally droopy and dragged down by making even the smallest effort
• Strong aversion to intercourse with total indifference to sexual partner

• Emotionally and mentally improved by vigorous exercise such as a power walking in the open air, or going to a exercise class
• Emotional symptoms are at their height after pregnancy, pre-menstrually and/or during the menopause

Head

• Dizziness on waking as a result of poor circulation or low blood pressure
• Migraines or headaches are aggravated by bright light, noise and changes of atmospheric pressure when a storm approaches. Nausea of migraine is made much more intense for coming into contact with the sight or smell of food
• Headaches are eased by contact with fresh air and having a sound sleep

Digestive

• Nausea and faintness develop quickly in response to skipping regular meals
• Eating a little temporarily eases nausea that has been triggered by low blood sugar levels
• Constipation with small, dry hard stools that are very slow and difficult to pass
• A sensation of a ball or lump or fullness remains in the rectum for a long time after passing a stool
• Severe pains after a bowel movement as a result of inflamed, bleeding haemorrhoids

Urination

• Persistent urge to pass water during the day and night, with a marked sense of pressure in the bladder
• Strong-smelling, discoloured urine with reddish-coloured sediment

Reproductive

- Complete mental, emotional and physical weariness and exhaustion pre-menstrually
- Severe mood swings, lethargy, irritability and scanty periods as part and parcel of pre-menstrual syndrome
- Morning sickness that is made noticeably more severe and distressing by delaying having something to eat (however small). As a result, it's greatly relieved by having a healthy, light snack at regular intervals
- Prolapse of the womb with an alarming feeling that everything is about to fall out of the pelvis
- Marked lack of enthusiasm for intercourse which can reach positive aversion. This is partly due to libido feeling flat as a pancake because of zero energy levels, and/or painful dryness of the vagina. This is most likely to become an issue leading up to, and after the menopause
- There may be lots of vaginal irritation and itching with a yellowish-green discharge
- Common extra menopausal symptoms include draining and exhausting hot flushes, plus heavy perspiration after making even the slightest effort

Sleep

- Drowsy by day but maddeningly wakeful at night
- Totally unrefreshed on finally waking when needing to face the day
- Perspiration and night sweats are especially troublesome and distressing during the night

Flushes and Fever

- Hot flushes alternate with heavy, distressing sweats. Although the flushes are severe, they don't result in any visible reddening of the skin
- Flushes move in an upward direction, from the legs to the upper parts of the body in an undulating, wave-like motion

Skin

- The appearance of skin conditions can be closely related to times of hormonal fluctuation. For instance, acne can pop up at puberty, eczema during the menopause and/or allergic rashes such as hives may be more likely to emerge before a period
- Irritated, itching skin feels more sensitive out of doors and is eased by warmth. But it can feel much worse for becoming overheated in bed
- A tendency to poor circulation leads to varicose veins and/or the skin taking on a mottled appearance

Muscles and Joints

- Dragging, heavy sensations that lodge in the lower back are eased by firm pressure. Back pain can be triggered or made more intense by a prolapse of the womb, or be associated with period pain cramps
- Heavy, weak sensation in the legs and specifically knee joints that have a tendency to 'give' when walking
- Resting makes the bruised tenderness in the joints generally more intense and distressing
- Pains in the knee joint with puffiness and swelling of the affected area that's more severe when going down stairs

SYMPTOMS ARE TRIGGERED OR MADE WORSE BY :

- Before, during or after a period
- Emotional responsibilities and demands
- Damp conditions
- Skipping regular meals
- Rest (this especially applies to joint pains)
- Sweating
- Being touched
- Making a mental effort

SYMPTOMS ARE EASED BY:

- Brisk exercise such as power walking, running or dancing
- Fresh air
- Eating small amounts often
- Firm pressure
- Warmth
- Elevating the legs

silica

Made from a homeopathic dilution of flint, this remedy is helpful in treating any of the following conditions: abcesses; acne; boils; dizziness; sinusitis; stress incontinence; stress-related problems (these may manifest as recurrent colds and minor infections, or poor skin, nail and hair quality); swollen glands; ulcers and wounds that are slow to heal and resolve themselves.

Core Features

- Very slow, insidiously-developing problems that come on over an extended period of time
- Symptoms of emotional and physical illness emerge slowly after going through traumatic, stressful or shocking life events
- Listlessness and tiredness with a noticeable inability to throw off minor infections involving the throat and glandular system. As a result, swollen glands and sore throats are a recurrent problem
- Wounds are slow to heal and become infected easily. Once they have healed, they have a tendency to leave stubborn scars
- Unstable circulation can lead to occasional flushes of heat, but chilliness is more a signature feature of those who benefit from this remedy

Emotional State

• Anxious, timid and significantly lacking in confidence and self-esteem. Due to an underlying conviction that taking on any challenge is likely to result in failure, there's a tendency to avoid any situations that may be potentially stressful or demanding
• Lack of confidence leads to an inability to reach a firm decision about anything important
• Phobias or compulsions can include a fear of sharp or pointed objects, triggering a phobia about injections. Rituals can also develop such as repeatedly checking doors are locked, or plugs of electrical items have been pulled out of sockets before leaving the house
• Irritable and emotionally short-fused when under stress and pressure
• Rigid, fixed ideas develop in response to pervasive insecurity and lack of confidence
• Easily startled and jumpy in response to loud noises when nervous, uptight and generally over-wrought
• Emotional and mental burn out leads to huge problems with mental focus and concentration. A hopeless depression can set in as a result of feeling so exhausted and overwrought
• When feeling well and energised those who do well with this remedy are capable of showing great conscientiousness with meticulous attention to detail. But when feeling ill, they're likely to lose any sense of drive, energy and motivation

Head

• Recurrent, bursting, intense headaches that begin at the nape of the neck, progressively affecting the whole of the head
• Headaches are aggravated by light, noise, exposure to cold and motion, while they are eased by firm pressure, wrapping the head up warmly, and heat in general

Respiratory (Throat, Nose and Chest)

• Persistent colds with lots of sneezing and an alternately dry and running nose
• The nose feels uncomfortably blocked with associated sinus congestion and tenderness
• Swollen and painful salivary glands with colds and sore throats
• Hoarseness with a dry cough that is made worse when speaking and drinking cool drinks
• Tickly, irritating sensation in the chest is soothed by warm drinks
• Coughing bouts are so severe they cause gasping and exhaustion when they're over

Digestive

• Nausea with aversion to water because it tastes unpleasant
• Abdominal discomfort and tenderness are eased by contact with warmth
• Recurrent or severe constipation that leads to significant difficulty in passing even a small stool. After a difficult bowel movement, sharp pains persist for a significant period of time
• Excruciatingly sensitive haemorrhoids or anal fissure

Reproductive

• Painful, irregular or absence of periods
• Irregular bleeding or 'spotting' between periods
• Smarting vaginal discharge that may look milky in colour

Skin

• Rapidly-infected skin that is very slow to heal. As a result, even the smallest wound or scratch can become inflamed or septic
• Recurring tendency to boils, abscesses, or carbuncles
• Scars are resistant to complete healing, and have a tendency to remain painful for a very long time

Muscles and Joints

• Cramping pains with weakness in the arms and legs
• Poor or sluggish circulation leads to a tendency to sensations of numbness, tingling, or 'pins and needles'
• Back pain is eased by warmth and made worse on first movement after rest

SYMPTOMS ARE TRIGGERED OR MADE WORSE BY:

• Exposure to dry, cold, windy weather
• Cold air
• Pressure
• Lying on painful areas
• During periods

SYMPTOMS ARE EASED BY:

• Summer weather
• Warmth applied locally
• Wrapping up warmly
• Resting

staphysagria

Made from a homeopathic dilution of the herb stavesacre, this remedy is helpful in treating: the after-pains of incised or lacerated wounds (especially those caused by surgical incision); baby blues (especially after a high-tech birth or section); bites and stings; cystitis; grief (especially where the angry phase of grieving has been suppressed or denied); joint pains; neuralgia; prostatitis; shingles and styes.

Core Features

• Symptoms that respond well to Staphysagria typically emerge as a consequence of anger, rage or indignation not being allowed it's natural expression
• Exquisite sensitivity on mental, emotional and physical levels, with hyper-awareness of pains that are stinging or sharp in their nature

- Often needed where there has been a history of emotional and/or physical abuse
- Symptoms often set in after any examination or surgical procedure that the patient views as invasive or a violation of privacy. This can happens as a result of medical investigations or treatments involving the genital area or radical surgery such as hysterectomy.
- Sensitive, shivery and chilly

Emotional State

- Very inwardly angry and resentful: broods and fumes inside rather than getting feelings off the chest at the time
- Trembles and shakes with the effort of suppressing anger. As a result of all of this emotional locking down, there's a tendency to become disproportionally upset and irritated by the mildest criticism
- Symptoms often emerge following events where grief, outrage, anger or humiliation are the appropriate responses, but where they have been suppressed
- Broods on past injustices, resentments and unfair treatment
- Poor, unrefreshing sleep pattern from persistent upsetting thoughts leads to apathy, low mood and listlessness during the day

Head

- Headaches with pains that lodge in the forehead. There may also be a general sensation of tightning, prickling or numbness in the head
- If dizziness is a problem, it's likely to be relieved when moving around and made more distressing when resting, lying down, or sitting down

Eyes

- A recurrent tendency to develop styes when run down. The margins of the eyelids feel itchy

Digestive

- Irritation and upset feeling in the stomach is made worse when smoking
- Burning pains and pressure in the stomach with retching
- Stomach upsets are triggered by feeling irritable and tense, or they may be made more troublesome by drinking cold water
- Stinging, burning, severe pains and sensitivity in haemorrhoids

Urination

- Cystitis that comes on after sex with constant, urgent need to pass water. Distressing pains linger for a long time afterwards
- Unpleasant sense of a drop of urine left behind in the urethra after passing water
- Urine looks dark-coloured and concentrated
- Stinging pains smart and burn when passing small amounts of urine

Reproductive

- Extra-sensitive vagina to sexual contact can move one of two ways: either this leads to a strong aversion to sex or a significantly increased libido
- Stinging pains or general heightened sensitivity in scars remains long after surgery
- Suppressed anger and resentment after a high-tech birth (especially involving Caesarian section), or episiotomy or hysterectomy can trigger feelings of depression as the anger is kept in
- Stitching pains and aching affect the scrotum and testicles
- Early onset of erectile dysfunction

Sleep

- Wakes from sleep feeling out of sorts, irritable, bad-tempered and generally unrefreshed by a night's rest
- As a result of poor sleep pattern and quality, there's a tendency to yawn constantly during the day, while finding it frustratingly difficult to drift into a deep sleep at night

Skin

- Lingering stinging pains and sensitivity in wounds and scars caused by lacerations that are very slow to heal
- Weepy, scaly skin that burns fiercely before and after scratching
- Noticeable and troublesome cycle or itch/scratch/itch, where having a good scratch does nothing to relieve irritation on the skin in the long-term. The itchy sensation moves from one location to another once one place has been scratched
- Distressing sensitivity with sharp, stinging pains during, and following, a bout of shingles

Muscles and Joints

- Stiff, aching joints that are made more painful and uncomfortable for touch and movement
- The longer joints are painful and stiff with well-established arthritis, they are likely to look mishapen as a result of developing bony nodules and outgrowths
- Pain and discomfort in the back is worse during the night and when resting
- The right shoulder may be especially affected, with pains being made much worse for movement

SYMPTOMS ARE TRIGGERED OR MADE WORSE BY:

- Suppressing feelings or anger, frustration, indignation and/or resentment
- Being subject to mental and emotional stress and strain
- Slight touch
- Sex
- Smoking
- In the early morning

SYMPTOMS ARE EASED BY:
- Resting
- Warmth
- Getting into a sound, refreshing sleep
- After eating breakfast

sulphur

Made from a homeopathic dilution of the element sulphur, this remedy can be helpful in treating: skin conditions such as acne, boils; catarrh; cradle cap; diarrhoea; eczema and/or psoriasis; German measles; hot flushes; measles; nappy rash; poor sleep pattern; swollen glands; thrush and wounds that are very slow to heal and tend towards easy infection.

Core Features
- Noticeable distress and discomfort when becoming overheated in stuffy, hot surroundings that provide little access to a fresh, cool air supply
- Burning, itchy skin that is made unbearably uncomfortable for becoming hot in bed, and /or after a bath or shower. The feet in particular are hugely heat-sensitive and where this remedy is well indicated, there's an established tendency to push them out of the bedcovers at night in an attempt to cool them off
- Hot, red skin that flushes up very quickly, with the skin around the eyelids, mouth, and wings of the nose looking red-rimmed and inflamed
- Low levels of stamina and vitality with a pattern of relapsing conditions. This is accompanied with a general state of exhaustion and lack of va-va-voom
- Blood sugar levels are easily made unstable, with a noticeable dip in energy that kicks in around mid-morning. When this happens, common features include

dizziness, weakness, and hunger pangs
- Signature discharges tend to be profuse, yellowish-green in colour, and offensive in consistency and odour
- Strong dislike of bathing or showering because it aggravates symptoms so much

N.B. The most important thing to bear in mind with respect to using this remedy is that it must be used very sparingly and with caution, especially in any situation where the skin is sensitive, itchy and inclined to erupt in response to very little provocation. As a result, although it is one of the most commonly-indicated remedies for treating itchy skin eruptions such as eczema, it has such as powerful de-toxing action that it is inadvisable to give it frequently over a long period of time. This is very important in order to avoid any aggravation of inflammation and itching.

Emotional State
- An inability to 'stay the distance' due to a deficiency of grit, persistence and staying power. As a result, there's a noticeable tendency to be unable to rise to, and meet challenges
- Touchy, irritable and self-absorbed with a tendency to philosophise about the smallest issues
- Sulks very readily when offended or feels criticised
- Beats around the bush endlessly, rather than being able to focus and take action decisively
- Unusual, contrasting combination of fastidiousness and messiness: the office may be in chaos, while the work that is produced from it is immaculate
- Weepy, withdrawn, anxious, brooding and depressed during periods and approaching menopause
- Obsessive ideas may develop

around religion, moral issues, or irrational anxieties about health and disease

Head
- Frequent bouts of dizziness that are likely to be especially severe as a result of standing for an extended length of time
- Light-headedness is associated with feeling sick and queasy, weakness and being short of breath
- Periodic headaches occur at weekends, or on holiday. These fall into the 'leisure sickness' category, and appear to be triggered by the release of stress during a period of relaxation
- Headaches are made more severe and distressing when out of doors or when stooping, and feel relieved by resting in moderate, constant temperature

Eyes
- Reddish, inflamed margins to the eyelids. The eyes may exude a yellow, crusty discharge
- Eyes feel itchy, red and burning

Respiratory (Throat, Nose and Chest)
- Recurrent, or slow-to-clear colds with persistent, mucus congestion in the nose
- The nose feels stuffed up and obstructed indoors and runs profusely when out of doors in the fresh, open air
- Dry, sore throat with a sensation of swallowing over a ball or lump in the throat. This stubbornly refuses to shift on swallowing of hawking
- Spasmodic, suffocative coughing bouts are relieved by contact with fresh, open air
- Wheezing and coughing episodes can alternate with flaring up of a skin condition such as eczema. When one is making its presence felt, the other is likely to be less in evidence

Digestive

- Hugely hungry with sudden hunger pangs and sinking in the stomach around mid-morning
- Sick, queasy feeling is made much worse for skipping meals
- Burning indigestion with violent belching
- Craving for fatty, spicy foods and alcohol, which makes indigestion more of a problem. Alternatively, there may be an aversion to eggs, milk, and fat
- Has to dash to the loo urgently in the early morning due to painless diarrhoea
- Diarrhoea alternates with constipation
- If diarrhoea continues for a while, this can produce problems with itching, rawness and soreness of the anus. This can cause a great deal of distress and discomfort in bed at night

Urination

- Burning, smarting pains that cause great distress on passing water
- Recurring kidney problems with general sensations of cold sweats, shivering and muscle aches when passing water

Reproductive

- Periods tend to be irregular with intermittent bleeding that stops and starts
- Delayed or early periods with dark flow that can vary between heavy and scanty in volume
- Hot flushes, shivering and faintness with menopausal symptoms
- Prolapse of the womb with a powerful bearing down sensation that is aggravated when standing
- Itching, irritation and burning discomfort in the vagina is noticeable during menopause when vaginal secretions become more scanty

Flushes and Fever

- Skin remains dry and hot during a flush, or it may sometimes break out into a sweat. This can turn into a heavy, clammy perspiration
- Although tending towards feeling so hot and flushed, there's a powerful dislike of being on overheated or uncomfortably draughty rooms
- The head is uncomfortably hot while the feet remain chilly, or the feet may join in and get burning hot
- Although very thirsty for cold drinks, sweat can be scanty

Sleep

- Wakes frequently around 3a.m. Once conscious, finds it difficult to drift back into sleep
- Jumps and starts just at the point of losing consciousness
- Finds it difficult to get up in the morning and has a powerful need to lie in. This is due to having an unrefreshing, unsatisfactory quality of sleep

Skin

- Itchy, inflamed, unhealthy skin that weeps, burns, or bleeds as a result of scratching
- Maddening, intense itching that feels aggravated by contact with heat and warmth in any form, especially the warmth of the bed, or bathing in warm or hot water
- Sensitive skin may also over-react and become very itchy and irritable after making contact with wool

Muscles and Joints

- Stiff, painful joints that are especially painful and immobile when getting up after sitting for a while
- Rapidly-developing numbness and tingling if a limb is kept in one position for any length of time
- Muscle pains and cramps are triggered by becoming heated in bed
- Back pains are made more intense by the slightest pressure or jarring movement

SYMPTOMS ARE TRIGGERED OR MADE WORSE BY:

- Contact with cold draughts that chill
- Becoming overheated
- In bed
- Standing for lengthy periods of time
- During and after washing
- On waking
- Mid-morning

SYMPTOMS ARE EASED BY:

- Stable, moderate temperatures
- Dry, warm weather

further reading

CHILDREN'S ISSUES

Homeopathic Medicine for Children and Infants
Dana Ullman
(Piatkus, 1992)

The Homeopathic Treatment of Children
Paul Herscu
(North Atlantic Books, 1991)

The Immunisation Decision: A guide for parents
Randall Neustaeder
(North Atlantic Books, 1990)

Nature's Child: guide, nourish and protect your child the gentle way
Leslie Kenton
(Ebury Press, 1993)

Vaccination and Immunisation: Dangers, delusions and alternatives
Leon Chaitow
(CW Daniel, 1987)

GENERAL HEALTH AND LIFESTYLE ISSUES

Authentic Woman: A guide to beauty, body and bliss
Leslie Kenton and
Susannah Kenton
(Vermillion, 2005)

Beauty Wisdom: The secret of looking and feeling fabulous
Bharti Vyas
(Thorsons, 1997)

Boost Your Energy Naturally
Beth MacEoin
(Carlton, 2003)

Boost Your Immune System Naturally
Beth MacEoin
(Carlton, 2001)

The Encyclopedia of Complementary Medicine: The definitive guide to the best treatment options for 200 health problems
Anne Woodham and
Dr David Peters
(Dorling Kindersley, 1997)

The Good Sleep Guide
Michael Van Straten
(Kyle Cathie, 1996)

How to be a Healthy Patient
Stephen Fulder
(Headway/Hodder and
Stoughton, 1991)

Natural Healing for Women
Susan and Frasier Curtis
(Horsons, 2003)

Natural Health for Women
Beth MacEoin
(Hamlyn, 2005)

Natural Medicine: A practical guide to family health,
Beth MacEoin
(Bloomsbury, 1999)

Simply Radiant: Practical techniques to turn back the years,
Bharti Vyas
(Thorsons, 1999)

The Total De-Stress Plan
Beth MacEoin
(Carlton, 2002)

Total Health: The essesntial family guide to conventional and complementary medicine
Dr David Peters
(Marshall publishing, 1998)

GENERAL TITLES ON HOMEOPATHY

**The Complete
Book of Homeopathy**
Michael Weiner and Kathleen Goss
(Bantam, 1982)

**The Complete Guide to
Homeopathy: The principles
and practice of treatment**
Dr Andrew Lockie and
Dr Nicola Geddes
(Dorling Kindersley, 1995)

**The Complete
Homeopathy Handbook**
Miranda Castro
(Macmillan, 1990)

**Everybody's Guide
to Homeopathic Medicines:
Taking care of yourself and
your family with safe and
effective remedies**
Dana Ullman and
Dr Stephen Cummings
(Gollancz, 1986)

**The Family Guide to Homeopathy:
The safe form of medicine for
the future**
Dr Andrew Lockie
(Elm Tree Books, 1989)

**Homeopathic Medicine for
the 21st Century**
Dana Ullman
(North Atlantic Books, 1988)

**Homeopathy for
Common Ailments**
Robin Hayfield
(Gaia, 1993)

Homeopathy for Everyone
Sheila and Robin Gibson
(Arcana, 1991)

**Homeopathy for Mother and
Baby: Pregnancy, birth and the
post-natal year**
Miranda Castro
(Macmillan, 1992)

**Homeopathy: Medicine
for the new man**
George Vithoulkas
(Thorsons, 1985)

**How to Use
Homeopathy Effectively**
Dr Christopher Hammond
(Element, 1991)

RESOURCES

**Ainsworths Homeopathic
Pharmacy**
Telephone: 00 44 (0) 1883 340332
or 00 44 (0)20 7935 5330
www.ainsworths.com

Helios Homoeopathy
Telephone: 01892 537254
Fax: 01892 546850
Email: pharmacy@helios.co.uk

Nelsons Homeopathic Pharmacy
Telephone:
Pharmacy 020 7629 3118
Telephone:
Mail order 020 7495 2404

HOMEOPATHIC ORGANISATIONS

The Society of Homeopaths
Telephone: 0845 450 6611
Fax: 0845 450 6622
www.homeopathy-soh.org

The Homeopathic Trust
For information on conventional
doctors who also use homepathy.
British Homeopathic Association
Hahnemann House
29 Park Street West
Luton LU1 3EE
Telephone: 0870 4443950
www.trusthomeopathy.org/contact.
html

HOMEOPATHIC SUPPLIES

**The Homeopathic Supply
Company**
Telephone: 01263 588788
Fax: 01263 588875
Email:
orders@homeopathicsupply.com
www.homeopathicsupply.com

index

homeopathy

285

homeopathy

acknowledgements

My warmest thanks must be extended to the following people who have all in their different capacities made this book a joy to work on. Caroline Taggart has been a delightful, enthusiastic and inspiringly intelligent editor to work with, while Vicki Murrell has engaged in the more detailed aspects of the editing process with impressive skill, patience and good humour.

As always, my deepest thanks go to my agent Teresa Chris without whose diligence, faith, energy and determination my writing career would have remained languishing in the wings. A crucially important role has also been played by Melanie Oxley from the Society of Homeopaths. Her willingness to give so freely of her time in providing an objective reaction to the first chapter, and the constructive nature of her reaction, were of enormous comfort when I felt too immersed in the text to see the proverbial wood for the trees. Many thanks are also due to John Morgan of Helios Pharmacy who made such encouraging and helpful suggestions in relation to chapter one, especially since these were given within an extremely challenging time frame.

On the personal front, mention must always be made of the pivotal role played by my husband Denis. Tirelessly helpful in trying to sort out yet another computer crisis of mine, always ready cast his eagle eye over the text as it was appearing, and ready with a cup of tea and a laugh when the going started to get too tough, writing would be quite another experience without him. Finally, where would I be without my own angel in furry, cat clothing Samantha? Without her purring, warmth and softness life would be a much more stressful business indeed.